# Cosmetic surgery

# → also available in the**facts** series

# the**facts**

# Cosmetic surgery

## NORMAN WATERHOUSE

Consultant Plastic and Aesthetic Surgeon,
Chelsea and Westminster Hospital,
London, UK

**OXFORD**
UNIVERSITY PRESS

# OXFORD
UNIVERSITY PRESS

Great Clarendon Street, Oxford OX2 6DP

Oxford University Press is a department of the University of Oxford.
It furthers the University's objective of excellence in research, scholarship,
and education by publishing worldwide in

Oxford New York

Athens Auckland Bangkok Bogotá Buenos Aires Calcutta
Cape-Town Chennai Dar-es-Salaam Delhi Florence Hong-Kong Istanbul
Karachi Kuala-Lumpur Madrid Melbourne Mexico-City Mumbai
Nairobi Paris São-Paulo Singapore Taipei Tokyo Toronto Warsaw

with associated companies in Berlin Ibadan

Published in the United States
by Oxford University Press Inc., New York

© Oxford University Press, 2008

The author is grateful for the illustrations provided by Anne Wadmore

First edition published 2008

British Library Cataloguing in Publication Data

Data available

Library of Congress Cataloging-in-Publication Data
Waterhouse, Norman.
  Cosmetic surgery / Norman Waterhouse.
    p. cm. — (The facts)
  Includes index.
  ISBN-13: 978–0–19–921882–0
1. Surgery, Plastic—Popular works. I. Title.
RD119.W38 2008
617.9′52—dc22                                                           2008003359

ISBN 978–0–19–921882–0

10 9 8 7 6 5 4 3 2 1

Typeset in Plantin
by Cepha Imaging Pvt. Ltd., Bangalore, India
Printed in Great Britain
on acid-free paper by
Ashford Colour Press, Gosport, Hampshire

To Margaret Hopkins, Peter Forrester, Cyrilla Chatfield, and the staff at the Wellington Hospital

# Foreword

Over recent years there has been an explosion in demand for and acceptance of cosmetic surgical and non-surgical procedures. These are procedures of choice, carried out to change appearance or to improve appearance. We live in a young world where people are living longer and remaining active to a much older age. Feeling fitter, more and more individuals want to keep looking fresh to make sure they enjoy life, happy with the way they look.

With surgery of choice it is even more important that patients fully understand the limitations of what can be achieved. We are bombarded with glossy images promoting improvements to sell surgical services, but there may not always be in the patients' interests. General practitioners are rarely consulted about cosmetic concerns, increasing the need for education about treatments.

This book outlines what can be achieved along with the limitations and indeed possible complications of surgery. It stresses the importance of finding the right surgeon, practising in the right environment, and the importance of being fully informed before embarking on treatments. These are sometimes life-changing decisions and must be properly considered, without hard-selling techniques.

Chapter by chapter, the main procedures are reviewed in a simple, easily understood way. The benefits and pitfalls are openly described to enable prospective patients to make more informed decisions about the options available. Whilst no book can replace a detailed consultation with a properly qualified surgeon this volume will educate and aid patients through the decision-making process to help ensure the right decisions are made.

Douglas McGeorge
President
British Association of Aesthetic Plastic Surgeons

# Contents

# 1

# Introduction

The specialty of plastic surgery aims to restore form and function to damaged, diseased, or abnormal tissues. It has no boundaries—a plastic surgeon might operate on a crushed hand, a cancer on the face, and a birth defect of the bladder in the same day.

Plastic surgery techniques have been practised since antiquity. Our modern methods of reconstructing the nose are similar to those described in India, 3000 years ago. The establishment of plastic surgery as a formal discipline is, however, a recent development, stimulated by the injuries of modern warfare. The rifles used in the First World War fired low-velocity bullets that were sufficient to cause tissue damage, splinter bone, and tear away flesh, but unlike high-velocity bullets, would not cause the energy waves that result in instant death. As a result many young men survived the war with appalling facial injuries. Independently, surgeons in France (Morestin), England (Gillies), and Germany (Esser), began to develop techniques and procedures to reconstruct the face. These included methods of moving skin and tissue from one place to another and replacing and building up tissue where it had been lost or damaged. The repair and reconstruction of damaged tissue was also applied to limb injuries and burns.

During the Second World War, Harold Gillies and Archibald McIndoe established a specialized plastic surgery unit at East Grinstead Hospital, to treat injured servicemen and civilians. Their work on the faces and hands of burnt airmen marked a significant advance in medicine that was accompanied by other enormous advances, such as the ability to transplant the cornea and restore sight. The so-called 'Guinea Pig Club' still exists today, and a dwindling number of surviving Royal Air Force pilots attest to the remarkable skills of these early pioneers.

Gillies and MacIndoe also had thriving private practices in which they carried out cosmetic surgery. Gillies, who was a meticulous and slow surgeon, was somewhat dismissive of MacIndoe's fast style and his interest in facial cosmetic surgery. Even in MacIndoe's biography it is not difficult to sense his reticence and guilt in pursuing his practice of cosmetic surgery. A quote from his wife records that she hoped that there would be 'no facelifters in this house'. This an important point because, until recently, there has been reticence from properly qualified plastic surgeons to acknowledge that they have a major interest in cosmetic surgery for fear that somehow this will be perceived as something trivial and not worthy of their skills. Despite this, it is a fact that almost all the major advances in cosmetic surgery have been discovered and developed by properly trained, established plastic surgeons.

There is often confusion as to the meaning of the terms cosmetic and plastic surgery. Plastic surgery involves the restoration of damaged or abnormal tissues to become as normal as possible. Cosmetic surgery describes the techniques used to improve or enhance tissues and structures that are normal—it is surgery to enhance or improve appearance. Plastic surgeons, even to this day, have often felt conflicted by their ability to reconstruct the abnormal and improve the normal. Cosmetic surgery has often been viewed as a disreputable use of surgical skills and, at worst, the province of 'quacks' and charlatans. In the USA, since the 1920s, there have been well-documented examples of unqualified surgeons offering and performing cosmetic surgery, frequently with disastrous results. Operations, including rhinoplasties (nose jobs) were not infrequently performed in hotel rooms! However, established, well-trained plastic surgeons appreciated that techniques to repair damaged structures in the face could be applied to a normal face to make it look better or younger. Early attempts at facelifting can be traced from the beginning of the twentieth century. These techniques were relatively simple and unsophisticated. Since then, enormous advances in knowledge, anatomy, technology, and techniques have revolutionized the treatment of facial surgery, both reconstructive and cosmetic. The same is true of breast surgery, liposuction, rhinoplasty, and almost all other forms of cosmetic surgery.

Cosmetic surgery was, until recently, a mysterious and secretive practice, reserved for a privileged minority of wealthy celebrities and film stars. A high-profile criminal might travel to Brazil for surgery to change his appearance and a film star might alter her nose but these options were rarely considered by the general population. How things have changed. Type cosmetic surgery into a major search engine and you will see that there are currently in the region of 11 million websites on the subject of cosmetic surgery. Cosmetic surgery articles feature on a weekly basis in newspapers, magazines and a variety of other forms of media. Advertisements for cosmetic surgery services can be found in almost every publication from cookery books to airline magazines. Television has had an even more specific impact in bringing the realities of cosmetic surgery to the public. The boundaries of obtrusiveness regarding medical procedures have been tested in the arena of cosmetic surgery, where we are now treated to graphic real-time operative sequences accompanied by commentaries by minor celebrities.

The interest in plastic surgery is global. The demand for plastic surgery in Iran, China, South East Asia, South Asia, and South America is enormous. Indeed, many of these countries are looking to position themselves as providers of cut-price cosmetic surgery for Western consumers who are encouraged to combine their surgery with holidays.

The third commonest reason to take out a personal loan in the UK, behind buying a car and house improvements, are to fund a cosmetic surgery procedure. The cosmetic surgery explosion probably reflects the fact that society has become more ageist and appearance conscious. It is frequently stated by potential patients that they seek cosmetic surgery in order to be competitive in the workplace, as well as for reasons of attractiveness. Some seek cosmetic surgery after major life events, such as bereavement or divorce.

The massive demand clearly has commercial implications and it is in this respect that cosmetic surgery is very different from other forms of surgical specialties. It would be almost inconceivable for cardiac surgery or neurosurgery to be marketed by businessmen with glossy adverts in the back of magazines. The so-called 'cosmetic industry' has mushroomed with no government interference or legislation. This has resulted in the general public being targeted by highly visible advertising for cosmetic surgery services.

These are often presented in an enticing and seductive manner using traditional marketing techniques. Many adverts will contain glossy photographs of naked or semi-naked beautiful bodies with idealized breasts, hips, thighs, and buttocks. Many of these adverts promote inducements, including interest-free loans and special 'two for one' offers. The nature of many of these adverts has been a cause for concern, in that patients seeking cosmetic surgery find it very difficult to distinguish between principled experienced providers and others who may make excessive and unrealistic guarantees for treatment by surgeons with limited experience and training.

Properly trained surgeons will have completed a training programme over many years to gain familiarity with the relevant surgical field. To improve on the normal, it is essential to be familiar with the treatment of the abnormal. The reason plastic surgeons are able to improve the size and shape of the breast is that they have a detailed knowledge base from treating the problems arising from surgery for breast cancer. These include reconstructing mastectomy defects after cancer surgery and restoring symmetry and volume for developmental breast anomalies.

Basic plastic surgery training places great emphasis on careful handling of body tissues to facilitate healing and minimize scar formation. This is of great importance in cosmetic surgery. As with all surgical disciplines, surgeons usually develop expertise in specific areas. Thus, a surgeon who specializes in breast surgery may not be an expert in facial surgery and vice versa. In certain areas, such as the eyelids or the nose, cosmetic surgeons may be from an ophthalmic or ENT (ear, nose, and throat) specialty.

Contemporary cosmetic surgery is now a highly sophisticated field and practitioners have a responsibility to be highly skilled in their particular domain. As with all surgical disciplines, cosmetic surgeons are encouraged to audit (analyse) their results and complications. Submitting these data is a mandatory requirement for all members of the British Association of Aesthetic Plastic Surgeons. They must demonstrate their participation in ongoing education and awareness of evolving surgical advances and techniques.

Potential consumers now have unparalleled access to high-quality information and an increasing sophistication of their treatment options and the skills of potential practitioners. However, choosing a doctor can still be a bewildering process, confronted with aggressive marketing by a variety of providers. The confusion as to who is a plastic surgeon and who is a cosmetic surgeon—some surgeons are both, and some neither—has implications for potential patients. If there is self-inflicted confusion among the medical profession as to what we should be called, it is hardly surprising that potential patients find claims and counter claims regarding expertise, accreditation, and qualification bewildering. At worst, it can appear that this is simply infighting between doctors scrabbling for the monetary rewards of cosmetic surgery.

There is no doubt that there is a huge discrepancy in the quality of service that is available for consumers of plastic surgery. Ideally, any potential patient should have access to a fully trained surgeon in an appropriate surgical specialty. This is usually plastic surgery, but could be ENT (for the nose) or ophthalmic surgery (for the eyes). Regrettably, this is not always the case. Indeed, some of the glossiest adverts for the most well-known surgical providers of cosmetic surgery may involve techniques such as counselling by a non-medical person who may be on commission to sell you surgery, enticing finance deals with 0% interest, no cooling off period, and not meeting your surgeon until the day of surgery. Your surgeon may be anybody recruited by the clinic. He or she may only be in the country for a short period of time and therefore not available for follow-up care or for correction of any complications.

Anyone considering cosmetic surgery would reasonably want to know:

- their surgeon is properly trained and experienced
- the hospital or clinic is properly staffed and equipped
- the range of results or success of a procedure
- the possible problems or complications
- the recovery time
- what aftercare is provided
- what complaint procedures are available.

Cosmetic surgery has now become an integral part of modern culture. Although there are an increasing number of surgical procedures in more and more surprising areas of the body, 10–12 operations account for 95% of all surgery. I have excluded genital surgery and fringe procedures of dubious value, and have restricted discussion of the enormous range of non-surgical cosmetic 'treatments' to Botox and fillers.

The following chapters aim to provide practical information and advice, designed for potential patients as well as a range of health professionals, including nurses, doctors, psychologists, and medical students.

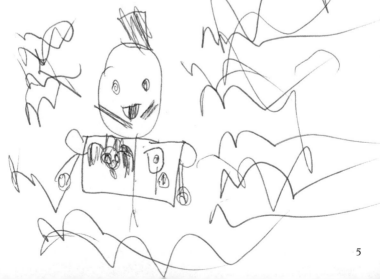

# 2

# Choosing a surgeon

For anyone considering a cosmetic procedure, the process of choosing a surgeon can be convoluted and confusing. Unlike most other branches of medicine, the traditional role of the general practitioner in recommending a specialist has been eroded in the field of cosmetic surgery. Many people feel that they shouldn't bother their GP for advice about cosmetic surgery because it is not 'serious' and may be a waste of their time. Regrettably, some GPs may indeed be unsympathetic or not know who to recommend.

It is now more usual to access information on providers from the internet or the advertisement sections of lifestyle magazines. Personal recommendations from friends who have undergone the procedure can be helpful and reassuring.

For many prospective patients, price is an important consideration. This ensures the popularity of heavily marketed commercial clinics offering the procedure at low cost and with a 'hard sell' approach. It should be understood that, in this competitive 'marketplace', the ability to make a profit from low-cost, high-volume operations means that savings are made from:

◆ employing surgeons who are willing to accept a low fee. These surgeons may not have appropriate expertise or qualifications in plastic surgery

◆ operating in surgical facilities or hospitals that do not provide an appropriate range of facilities.

At the present time, the UK government is examining the regulation of cosmetic surgery and is likely to impose tighter controls on surgeons' qualifications and expertise, the facilities and standards of hospitals, and an adherence to a code of conduct regarding marketing and advertising.

What then, should a prospective patient look for to ensure a high level of professional care and expertise? For anyone needing cardiac, gynaecological, neurosurgery, or orthopaedic surgery, it is taken for granted that their surgeon:

◆ has completed a surgical training programme in the specialty

◆ has passed examinations and assessments to demonstrate their knowledge and competence

◆ has acquired experience in treating patients with similar conditions

◆ will provide independent and professional guidance as to your suitability for surgery

◆ will give honest and clear information as to the possible risks and complications

◆ will carry out treatment in an accredited, properly equipped, and staffed hospital or clinic

◆ will provide seamless aftercare during the patient's recovery.

As a general guide, anyone considering cosmetic surgery should ensure the surgeon is qualified. This means that he or she has successfully completed a surgical training programme and passed professional examinations in plastic surgery or another relevant discipline (ophthalmic, ENT, maxillofacial, or breast surgery). They will then be awarded a CCST (Certificate of Completion of Surgical Training) and be entered on the Specialist Register, held by the General Medical Council.

The vast majority of surgeons with this qualification will be appointed as Consultants in an NHS hospital. Within this group, many will have particular training and expertise in specific areas or operations, including cosmetic surgery.

Interest and expertise in cosmetic surgery may be determined by:

◆ membership of a specialist association; for example, the British Association of Aesthetic Plastic Surgeons or The British Association of Oculoplastic Surgeons

◆ their stated specialist interest in cosmetic surgery

◆ their record of teaching and research in the field of cosmetic surgery

◆ their participation in national audit initiatives (this means that their results and complications have been produced and reviewed)

◆ personal recommendations from friends who have undergone the procedure can be helpful and reassuring.

It is important to know that possession of the qualification 'FRCS' and presence on the specialist register of the General Medical Council do not guarantee the above!

## The consultation

At any initial consultation with a cosmetic surgeon, any potential patient should expect:

◆ to be seen by the surgeon who would personally perform their procedure

◆ to be able to enquire as to the surgeon's training and qualifications

◆ a thorough enquiry as to their medical history, including medication, allergies, previous operations, reaction to anaesthesia, and any past or present psychological or psychiatric problems

◆ an exploration of their goals and expectations of surgery

◆ a thorough clinical examination, often including photography

◆ an honest and frank explanation as to their suitability for surgery, including the recovery time and likelihood of complications

- the opportunity to view photographs of previous patients' results from similar procedures

- the option of speaking to previous patients who have undergone similar procedures

- to know how frequently the surgeon performs the procedure

- to be offered written information on the procedure

- to be offered a second consultation after a period of reflection

- to know that the operation will be performed in an accredited, properly equipped, and staffed hospital

- to know what happens if there are complications and whether this will involve further cost.

A potential patient should not:

- be seen by a 'counsellor' or 'advisor' and given advice as to their suitability for surgery

- be offered inducements to proceed with surgery. These include discounts for immediate booking and payment of deposits.

For many considering cosmetic surgery, the cost can be prohibitive. This has encouraged the growth of 'surgical tourism' to providers of cosmetic surgery in a variety of countries in Europe and beyond; these include, Poland, Tunisia, and South Africa. While it is accepted that appropriately trained and skilled surgeons are often available, the decision to seek treatment abroad should be carefully considered.

- Payment in advance makes it difficult to decide not to proceed with surgery.

- There is no knowledge of the skill and experience of the surgeon or the anaesthetist.

- There is no knowledge of the facilities of the hospital.

- There may be problems with communication and language.

- There is no prospect of aftercare or treatment of any complications.

- There is little prospect for redress or complaint in the event of unsatisfactory treatment.

# Conclusions

Cosmetic surgery is a surgical specialty, demanding a high level of training, experience, and skill. However, its popularity and financial reward has attracted many doctors, from various backgrounds and with limited experience, to promote their services in this arena. Potential patients should be able to access reliable information to ensure they are treated by appropriately trained and experienced practitioners who will provide independent professional and skilled care. Caring for anyone undergoing a surgical procedure requires a team approach. This demands experience and skills from plastic surgery nurses, theatre staff, and anaesthetists.

# 3
# Breast augmentation

## ➔ Key points

♦ The decision to have breast implants has long-term implications.

♦ Your surgeon should offer lifelong follow-up care.

♦ Breast implants do not cause cancer or autoimmune diseases.

♦ Not all breast implants are the same. Insist on the highest quality with a lifetime guarantee.

Cosmetic breast surgery consistently ranks as one of the most frequently requested procedures by women. Over a quarter of a million women in the USA and 30 000 in the UK undergo breast augmentation every year. Although the primary motivation is a desire for larger breasts, many women are looking for a more attractive breast shape or restoration for more youthful breasts after childbirth and breastfeeding.

The benefits of breast augmentation include increased confidence and self-esteem, a greater sense of femininity and sexuality, and the ability to wear a range of clothes, swimwear, and lingerie. The vast majority of women are fearful that their implants will be obvious and unnatural. The most frequently expressed ideal is for a full-breasted look that is in proportion to their bodies. Implanted breasts should ideally look like breasts, feel like breasts, and move like breasts. Achieving a natural result depends on selecting a suitable and sensible size of implant and having enough breast tissue to conceal the implant.

Any woman considering breast augmentation should know that:

♦ a scar is inevitable (under the breast, around the nipple or in the armpit) (see Figure 3.1 overleaf)

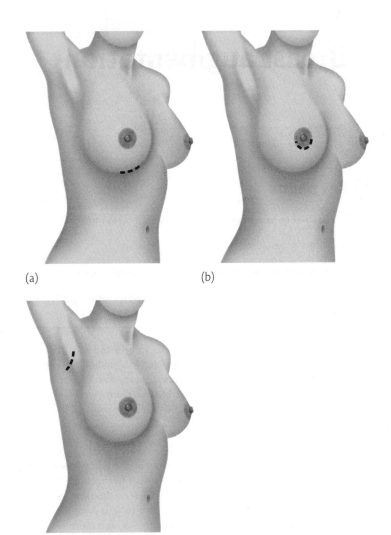

(a)

(b)

(c)

**Figure 3.1** (a) The scar under the breast. (b) The scar around the areolar. (c) The scar in the axilla.

- a technique exists for placing the scar around the umbilicus (belly button) this approach is complicated and carries a significant risk of complications

- the operation may result in decreased nipple sensation

- the implants may need to be replaced after 10–15 years

- the implant edge may be palpable or even visible, particularly in a thin patient with little natural breast tissue

- the implants may be firmer than a non-implanted breast

- the operation requires a general anaesthetic and an overnight stay in hospital

- mammography may be more difficult to interpret.

## Assessment

Suitable candidates for surgery must be advised on the types and size of implant that are appropriate to meet their expectations. This decision is based on many factors specific to individual circumstances, including:

- existing size, shape, and volume of the breast

- the anatomy of the chest, including muscle size and tone

- age and parity

- significant breast asymmetry (difference in size between the breasts)

- harmony with the waist and hips

- the patient's request.

---

### Implant placement

The implant can be placed under the breast tissue in a 'subglandular' pocket or under the pectoralis major chest muscle in a 'submuscular' pocket.

- The submuscular approach may involve more discomfort and a slightly longer recovery period. However, it produces a more natural

---

appearance in the upper pole of the breast and has a lower incidence of capsular contracture (see Figure 3.2 below).

♦ The subglandular approach offers a quicker recovery and is more suitable when the nipple is in a lower position on the breast. Implants placed in this way may be more visible and 'obvious'.

## Silicone issues

During the 1990s, doubt was cast on the safety of silicone implants. Suggestions that they may be responsible for an increase in the incidence of diseases such as arthritis, chronic fatigue syndrome (ME), and even cancer, generated a high level of anxiety in women with implants and deterred many from seeking surgery.

Until recently, silicone implants were banned from use in the USA for cosmetic augmentation, although they were still allowed for women undergoing breast reconstruction after mastectomy. Surgeons in America continued to meet the

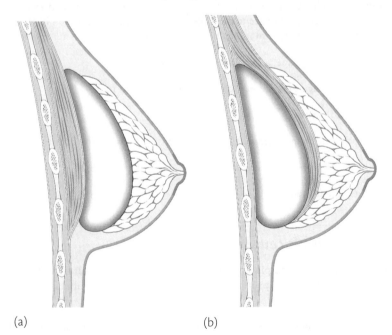

(a)                              (b)

**Figure 3.2** The breast in profile with an implant (a) above and (b) below the pectoralis muscle.

demand for augmentation by using implants filled with saline (salt water). The silicone embargo also stimulated the development of other types of implants such as those filled with soya oils.

The anxieties generated by the silicone issue prompted a plethora of research studies to determine the evidence of proposed risks to women's health. After several years, the consensus of independent studies found no evidence to suggest that silicone was responsible for any of the conditions under scrutiny. However, as a result of the studies, it has been recommended that women undergoing augmentation should consider exchanging their implants after 10–15 years in order to avoid implant rupture, which might occur after this time.

The rehabilitation of silicone gel-filled implants has been welcomed by plastic surgeons as most believe that they produce the most natural results. Manufacturers of breast implants (prostheses) have to comply with exacting directives on quality and safety. Technological advances have reduced the likelihood of implant leakage and reduced the problem of 'hardening' or 'encapsulation' of the implanted breast. At the present time, silicone implants are considered to be appropriate for use as medical devices with excellent safety profiles and few risks to women's health (http://www.silicone-review. gov.uk). Some implant manufacturers offer a lifetime warranty, which includes replacement of implants in the event of rupture and encapsulation. (http:// www.mentorcorp.com, http://www.allerganandinamed.com).

Advances in implant technology have resulted in the development of a range of products that vary in shape, consistency, and design and they may contain a range of silicone polymers that vary in texture and viscosity. Until recently, all implants were round and varied in 'projection'. The development of the 'anatomical' or 'shaped' implant offers surgeons and patients the option of an implant design that simulates a more natural 'teardrop' shape. However, the round implant is still very popular and produces excellent results. There are pros and cons of both types, which should be clearly explained during the consultation process.

## The consultation

Every woman presenting for a consultation should expect:

- the consultation to be with an appropriately qualified and experienced surgeon who will be carrying out any agreed procedure

- not to see a 'counsellor', nurse, or paramedical practitioner

- not to be induced or encouraged to proceed with surgery by financial offers

- not to 'sign up' to surgery or place a deposit at the first visit or before the consultation has taken place

- the consultation to include a thorough enquiry as to your medical history, general health, and current medication

- a thorough review of your breast health, including age of menarche, pregnancies, breastfeeding, previous breast lumps and family history of breast cancer, and use of oral contraceptives and hormone replacement therapy (HRT).

- a thorough breast examination in the presence of a chaperone (you may want to be accompanied by a friend or family member who should be welcome to observe the consultation and examination)

- an honest opinion as to your suitability for the procedure and an explanation of the various options available

- a discussion of the potential complications of the procedure and whether you are at particular risk

- the opportunity for you to ask questions of the surgeon including specific enquiries as to his/her qualifications and expertise; you should be able to view photographs of his or her results (most surgeons will be happy to put you in touch with a previous patient who had a similar procedure)

- to be offered a second consultation after a period of reflection

- a second consultation that includes an opportunity to determine the size of the implant (this can be assessed by placing different trial implants in a sports bra and viewing the effect with a range of clothing)

- to have photographs taken

- to be given a quote for the cost of the procedure, including the surgical, anaesthetic, and hospital fees

- to know of any additional costs resulting from any complications or need for revisional or corrective procedures

- to receive an information pack for further reading.

Most healthy women with small breasts may be suitable candidates for breast augmentation. They can expect an increase in confidence and self-esteem, although this should be balanced against the limitations and long-term implications of surgery. A major consideration for a successful outcome is the position of the nipple on the breast. With age or after breastfeeding, the breast may become empty, saggy, or droopy. Often, this also results in the nipple position being lower on the breast. If the nipple is only a little lower, augmentation may help to lift them. However, if the nipple is very low, a straightforward augmentation will not produce an attractive result. In these circumstances, the nipple may need to be lifted. This procedure is called a mastopexy and usually involves more scars (see Chapter 5).

Most women have breasts of slightly different sizes. When there is significant difference in size between the breasts (asymmetry), breast augmentation may be more complex and involve different implant sizes and additional adjustments.

Implant surgery may be inappropriate for women with:

◆ a family history of breast cancer. If you have a first-line relative with breast cancer, guidance should be offered to explain your cancer risk management

◆ previous breast pathology (mastitis, mastalgia, or multiple breast lumps)

◆ coexisting medical conditions such as autoimmune disorders, diabetes, and bleeding disorders

◆ dependence on optimal function of chest musculature (such as athletes)

◆ previous history of psychiatric disorders

◆ medication that thins the blood.

Breast implants may not produce a pleasing result for women with:

◆ ptotic (droopy) breasts (see Chapter 5, Mastopexy)

◆ tuberose breasts (narrow, conical breasts often with a large areola)

◆ very thin chest skin

◆ a tendency to form bad scars.

## The operation

Once you have decided to proceed, you should receive additional information relating to preparation for surgery. This will include advice on restrictions on medication, such as aspirin and anti-inflammatory drugs, and the use of arnica to reduce bruising postoperatively. You may be required to have a blood test to screen for the presence of anaemia or infections. You will normally be expected to attend the hospital for admission in the morning, having had nothing to eat or drink since 12.00 o'clock the previous night. The operation usually takes between 1 and 2 hours.

◆ Before surgery, you will be visited by your surgeon and an anaesthetist. Some marking of the breast may be performed.

◆ After the operation, you will be taken to a recovery ward where specialist nurses will monitor you through the period immediately after waking from the anaesthetic.

◆ You will normally be returned to the ward after an hour or so.

◆ You may have drains (small tubes) from your chest connected to plastic bottles. These are to allow the removal of any blood or fluid from the site of the operation. Usually, they are removed the following morning.

◆ Pain relief will be monitored by the anaesthetist.

◆ Discharge from hospital is usual the day after surgery. You will receive specific instructions and guidance on aftercare and have follow-up appointments provided.

◆ You should also have telephone numbers of members of the surgical team or hospital ward to contact if you have questions or concerns.

## Postoperatively

It is normal for the breasts to be swollen and the skin a little shiny—the swelling resolves after 7–10 days; however, further softening of the breasts may continue for some months. The nipples may be numb or occasionally hypersensitive for a week or two after the operation. Occasionally, tenderness and sensitivity in the nipples may be severe enough to require the placement of a plaster or dressing over the nipples for a week or two. Numb nipples usually recover sensation after a few weeks or even months.

You should wear a well-fitting sports bra night and day for at least 2 weeks and avoid rigorous exercise, lifting, and sexual activity for about 4 weeks. Stitches will be removed between 7 and 10 days and you will be advised as to management of your scars. This may include moisturizing and/or the use of a specific gel to apply to the scar to speed up healing.

Usually, you will be given a course of antibiotics when you leave the hospital. Take the whole course!

## Follow-up care

You should be reviewed by your surgeon after 6 weeks and again at 6 months; however, you should have access to your surgeon in the event of any concerns or problems arising in between appointments. Many surgeons offer a regular review appointment on an annual basis.

## Complications of breast augmentation

Complications can be subdivided into 'early' or 'late'. Early complications are rare. The most significant and common event is the development of a 'haematoma'. This occurs when bleeding into the breast quickly produces a swollen, painful breast. Haematomas are rare, occurring in about 2% of all cases. Treatment is always required and involves a return to the operating theatre to drain off the blood and stop any bleeding blood vessels. Once prompt effective management has been delivered, no serious long-term problems will occur, although the affected breast may be swollen for a few weeks.

Infection after augmentation is a feared but very rare complication. When it occurs, the breast will typically become hot, painful, and swollen. You may feel generally unwell and have a temperature. If an infection of this type occurs, there is usually no alternative but to remove the implant and commence a course of antibiotics. The implant can usually be reimplanted after an interval of a few months.

Rarely (less than 1%), nipple sensation may be reduced or even lost after augmentation.

### Late complications

These problems may only become apparent after a period of months or even years. They include:

- visibility or palpability of the implant through the skin

- rupture of the implant

- capsular contracture.

## What is capsular contracture?

Since the procedure began in the 1960s, the most frequent problem experienced by women with implants has been hardening or 'encapsulation' of the breast. The body will normally respond to the presence of an implant (or any other prosthetic medical device) by producing a thin layer of scar tissue around the implant. If this scar tissue is excessive, the implant becomes hard and unyielding to touch. The implant may become distorted or obviously round. Pain and discomfort may also occur. Treatment of capsular contracture can be difficult and the problem may recur.

Happily, the problem of capsular contracture is now much less frequent. This is largely due to advances in implant technology and design. Most implants are now 'textured'. This means that the implant surface is rough or 'stippled' and it seems that this reduces the ability for thick scar tissue to develop.

The problem can still occur (significant capsules may develop in 5% of cases) and may require either revisional surgery or removal of the implants.

## Treatment of capsular contracture

This may include:

- the surgeon squeezing the breast to tear the capsule (this may be painful and produce pain and swelling; the practice has been largely abandoned as it may cause implant rupture)

- an open procedure to release the capsule surgically

- the use of external ultrasound energy on the breast

- medical treatment with zafirlukast (Accolate), a drug normally used for asthma (some surgeons do not offer this option as there is a risk of liver damage with this drug).

 FAQ

Q1 Can I fly? Do implants explode on aeroplanes?

A There is no risk of implants exploding on aeroplanes and it is completely safe to fly. You can also scubadive to 30 metres without any problems!

Q2  Can I breastfeed with implants?

A  Implant surgery does not interfere with the breast anatomy for lactation and breastfeeding should not be affected.

Q3  Will it increase my risk of developing breast cancer?

A  No. Studies have actually shown that women with implants have a lower chance of developing the disease than women without implants. This lower risk is not due to the implants but because small-breasted women are less likely to develop cancer.

Q4  How long will I need off work?

A  Most women take 2 weeks off work although they can usually drive after 10 days and can manage gentle activity after a week. Women with implants placed on top of the pectoralis muscle usually recover quicker.

Q5  When can I go back to the gym?

A  Normally, it takes 3 or 4 weeks before a full range of gym activity can be resumed. Training of chest wall and arm muscles may require 6 weeks. Vigorous walking may be resumed after 10 days. Sexual activity should be avoided for 2 weeks and the breasts should be treated very gently for a further 3 weeks.

Q6  How long will my implants last?

A  Current advice to women is that the implants may need to be replaced after 10–15 years. However, it is likely that this is a cautious recommendation and they may in fact last for twice or three times as long.

## Alternatives to implants

There has been considerable interest in the options for increasing breast size without the need for breast implants or even any surgical procedure. In the future, gene therapy and the use of stem cells to grow breast tissue are exciting possibilities. At the present time, there are two realistic options for augmentation without implants.

## Vacuum suction expansion

Recent research in the USA has suggested that breast tissue can be increased if the breasts are exposed to continuous tension. It has been known that cell growth can be stimulated by external forces such as stretching. This is dramatically demonstrated by the use of 'lip plates' to stretch the mouth and weights attached to the ear lobes.

This biological phenomenon has been explored in relation to breast tissue and commercially developed by the BRAVA® system. The technique requires that a chest device is worn, connected to a vacuum system. This applies a constant tension to the breast, enclosed within the device. This must be worn for a minimum of 10 weeks and tension applied for as many hours in the day as possible. Practically, this requires the system to be used overnight and at home.

A demonstrable increase in breast size has been established; however:

- The system is cumbersome and requires constant use for a long time.

- The increases in breast size are modest, at best giving an increase of one cup size.

- After discontinuing the treatment, the breasts often revert to their pre-treatment volume.

## Fat transfer

The use of fat injections is discussed in other chapters (see Chapters 8 and 13 for more on facelift and fillers). Modern methods of preparing and injecting fat have increased the reliability of permanent survival. Fat transfer has an undoubted benefit in the face to replace lost volume and fill out lines and hollow areas. More recently, there has been considerable interest in using fat transfer to increase breast size. The concept is extremely attractive as it offers the prospect of a more natural way of augmenting the breast using one's own tissue.

However, there are some issues and anxieties regarding the use of fat transfer in the breast. It is possible that interpretation of mammograms may be difficult. If injected fat does not survive, non-viable cells may become calcified and possibly mimic cancerous changes.

## 🛈 Patient's perspective

Allison is 24 years old. She has two older sisters. Ever since puberty, she has been self-conscious about her small breasts. Both her sisters have 'C' cup breasts. She has a 'double A' cup and barely needs to wear a bra. This makes her feel unfeminine and unattractive. Buying clothes is difficult. She has never bought a bikini.

Breast augmentation has been on her mind for as long as she can remember and she is now able to afford the cost of surgery. Allison had exhaustively researched the subject and sought a reputable surgeon in her area. She found several clinics and surgeons offering breast augmentation and drew up a shortlist of three. All of these had websites with factual information on the procedure and representative pictures of pre- and postoperative results.

In the event, Allison decided to proceed after her first consultation. She liked the surgeon and the practice nurse and felt comfortable with the clear explanation of all the issues and possible long-term consequences, including the possibility of having to have the implants replaced after 15 years.

She had been asked to attend the consultation with a sports bra, of the size she thought she wanted. Based on the similarity of her body size and shape with that of her sisters, Allison chose a 'C' cup bra.

After the surgeon examined her breasts, she spent some time trying out different implants placed inside the sports bra. With the help of a full-length mirror, she was able to picture the effect of different sizes. She was pleased to find that her instincts were right and liked the 'C' cup size best. It seemed to suit her body. Allison was also shown a number of different types of implant. As well as the round shape, there was also the option of using an 'anatomical' or teardrop-shaped implant. Also, some implants were designed to give more projection or 'fullness'.

At first, she felt a little confused by the options available; however, the surgeon and the nurse carefully explained the various advantages and disadvantages. The surgeon explained that for her shape, a round implant would give an excellent full-breasted appearance that would suit her and appear natural.

Allison was offered a second consultation after a period of reflection and felt so confident that she decided to proceed and made a provisional booking for the operation immediately. She was given an extensive information sheet that included details of recovery times and possible complications. She was told that she would receive a letter from the anaesthetist regarding any anxieties or questions she might have regarding her general anaesthetic.

As the date for surgery approached, the practice nurse telephoned Allison and asked if she was sure she did not want to come for another consultation. The nurse also went over a few practical details regarding the admission to hospital.

The night before surgery, Allison went through the checklist she had been given by the practice nurse. Into her overnight bag went toiletries, a change of clothes and, most importantly, a 'C' cup sports bra. She arrived at the hospital at 7.00 AM, unsure whether the feeling in her stomach was hunger (no breakfast!) or anxiety. She was shown to her room and asked to change into a surgical gown. Her temperature, pulse and blood pressure were all recorded by the ward nurse as normal.

The anaesthetist came to see her and reviewed her medical history. He listened to her heart and lungs with a stethoscope. He then explained how she would feel afterwards and what pain medication would be prescribed. As Allison was going to have her implants placed under the pectoralis muscle, she knew that her chest area would feel sore for a few days. He had sent Allison a questionnaire to fill in a week before her surgery. When she filled it in, she had asked if she could have a 'premed' (this is medication to relieve anxiety and induce a relaxed sleepy feeling while waiting to go down to the operating theatre). Her premed was given after the surgeon came to see her. She needed to be alert to sign her consent form for surgery!

After the premed, her memory of the trip down to the operating theatre and waking up after surgery all seemed a bit of a blur. Before she realized it, her surgeon and anaesthetist were visiting her in her room and her operation was over. Although she did not take a proper look, she was overjoyed to see that she was wearing her sports bra and filled it snugly! The morning after surgery, Alison had been discharged home following removal of her drains. Although she did feel some discomfort, the painkillers were very helpful for the first few days. In fact, Allison did not get to see her new breasts properly for 10 days. This was when she returned to the surgeon's clinic where the practice nurse removed her tiny stitches under the breast.

Although they were still swollen and the skin was tight and shiny, Alison was thrilled. At last, she thought, I have breasts like my sisters!

Six weeks later, her new breasts were much softer and looked very natural. Her nipples had been a little tender and sensitive for a few weeks but had now returned to normal. Alison had treated herself to some new lingerie and swimwear, including her first ever bikini!

The novelty of her new shape still hadn't worn off. Every night, she looked at her body in her bedroom mirror with delight. She was so pleased that the surgery had matched her hopes. Six months after surgery, the scars under the breasts had begun to fade and Alison could hardly remember her pre-surgery shape.

# 4

# Breast reduction

## ➲ Key points

◆ Candidates for breast reduction must accept the inevitability of scars on the breasts.

◆ Breast reduction is one of the most popular and successful procedures in the field of cosmetic surgery.

◆ A mammogram should be performed on all women over the age of 45 before surgery.

It is ironic that a desire for bigger breasts is one of the commonest requests for cosmetic surgery and yet, for many women, large breasts can be a source of misery. Heavy large pendulous breasts can be the source of many physical and practical problems. They are heavy and may cause postural problems, including back and shoulder pain. Even the strain on a bra strap produces grooves in the shoulders. Exercise such as running or swimming is often impossible, which may predispose to general weight gain.

Large breasts are often a source of embarrassment and attract unwanted attention and comments. Disproportionately large breasts can limit choice of clothing. In the skinfolds underneath the breasts, the skin often becomes irritated and inflamed and may predispose to fungal infections. More rarely, the skin and breast tissue may develop sores or ulcers due to a reduced blood supply. Few women regard their large breasts as attractive. They go to great lengths to disguise them and often become round shouldered. Wary of drawing attention to themselves, many feel they become shy and passive, which may limit their potential in the workplace as well as socially. There are psychological as well as physical consequences.

Most women who develop large breasts have a genetic predisposition and there is often a family history. Pregnancy and weight gain may also be factors. There is also a rare condition called 'gigantomastia' where enormous breast size is a consequence of sensitivity to oestrogen.

Occasionally, asymmetry of the breasts may be pronounced, with one breast much larger than the other.

The range of problems experienced by women with large breasts leads many to seek surgery. Breasts before reduction are shown in Figure 4.1.

# What is breast reduction?

Breast reduction is a surgical procedure that reduces the size and volume of the breast. There are a number of different techniques that may be used according to individual needs and surgeon's choice. These include:

### Breast liposuction

In some circumstances, the breast can be reduced by liposuction alone. This option is attractive as it produces minimal scars and recovery is quick. However, it is only effective when a significant amount of the breast tissue is composed of fat. Glandular breast tissue is firmer and cannot be easily removed by suction. The other limitation is that after significant reduction by liposuction, the breast may become droopier and lax as no skin has been removed.

Sometimes liposuction can be useful as part of a formal breast reduction, to remove fat in the lateral part of the breast extending into the axilla (armpit).

### Surgery

All formal breast reduction operations involve removal of breast tissue and reshaping the breast. This almost always includes the need to remove excess skin. Traditionally, breast reduction results in scars, which are around the areola (the brown skin around the nipple), a vertical scar down to the base of the breast and a transverse scar in the fold under the breast (Figure 4.2). This scar pattern is often referred to as an 'inverted T' or 'anchor'.

In recent years, newer techniques of breast reduction have been developed, aimed at reducing the extent of the scars. These include a 'periareolar' approach where the scar is limited to the areola (Figure 4.3) or the so-called 'vertical scar' operation, which avoids the horizontal scar under the breast (Figure 4.4).

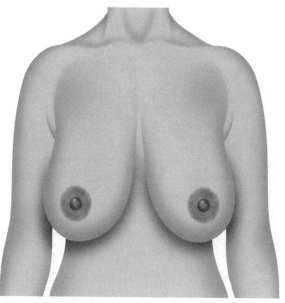

**Figure 4.1** Breasts before reduction.

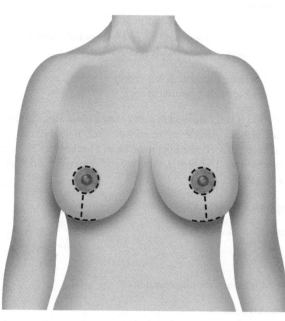

**Figure 4.2** Breasts with 'inverted T' or 'anchor' scars.

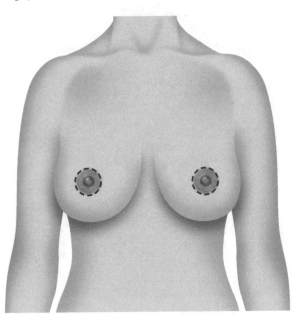

**Figure 4.3** Breasts with periareolar scars.

These procedures are popular and successful, but may not be practical if the breasts are very large or if the skin is thin and lax.

The aim of a breast reduction is not simply to reduce the size of the breasts but to achieve an attractive natural shape.

Breast reduction is still a significant surgical operation, although it has become safer and less daunting in recent years. Advances in anaesthesia and surgical techniques have reduced the operating time, bleeding, and swelling with a shorter recovery period. However, there are still several potential complications of surgery, which include:

- haematoma (bleeding into the breast after surgery)

- infection

- fat necrosis

- loss or reduction of nipple sensation

- thick, raised scars

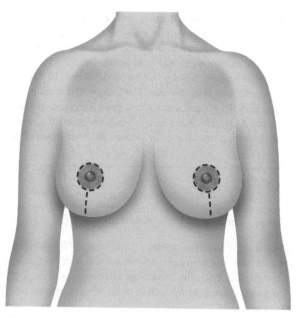

**Figure 4.4** Breasts with vertical scar patterns.

- nipple necrosis

- asymmetry.

Complications are rare but may be greater in specific circumstances. Breast reduction may not be suitable for:

- heavy smokers

- diabetic patients

- overweight or obese patients

- people with a known tendency to form poor scars

- a history of blood clotting problems

- a strong family history of breast cancer (many surgeons recommend that the tissue removed during breast reduction is sent for microscopic analysis in any woman over the age of 40).

Any woman undergoing breast reduction should be generally healthy and well. She should accept that the trade-off for smaller breasts will result in permanent scars on the breasts. The operation is usually performed under general anaesthetic and involves an overnight stay in hospital. Drains are often placed and removed a day after surgery. Stitches are removed after 7–10 days and a sports bra is usually worn for at least 2 weeks. The scars will gradually fade for up to 2 years after surgery. To minimize the scars, many surgeons encourage the use of a locally applied gel, which has been shown to improve scar remodelling. Some degree of scarring may always be evident after reduction surgery.

## ❓ FAQ

Q1 At what age can I have a breast reduction?

A It is possible to have this surgery at any age. Many women opt for surgery in their late teens or early twenties. It is also often requested after completing a family. Increasing discomfort and back pain may lead to surgery being performed in older women, sometimes in their sixties or seventies.

Q2 Can I breastfeed after surgery?

A In theory, there is no reason why women cannot breastfeed after surgery. Surgery does not disrupt the milk ducts' connection to the nipple.

Q3 Is it permanent?

A For the most part, the results of reduction surgery are permanent. However, when breast reduction is performed in young women, there is the possibility of recurrent growth of the breasts during and after subsequent pregnancy.

Q4 When can I return to work?

A Usually, return to work is possible after 2 weeks. However, return to vigorous exercise and sport should be restricted for 4 weeks. Even then, support with a sports bra is advisable.

Q5 Are there different operations?

A Yes. Reduction in breast volume can be achieved in different ways. Sometimes this is possible with liposuction. This can be performed with very small scars and recovery is rapid. Most techniques involve a formal reduction of breast tissue and skin. Depending on the degree and individual factors, the resultant scars may vary from a scar around the areola to additional scars from the nipple areola complex down to the base of the breast and a transverse scar in the fold at the base of the breast.

Q6 What are the complications?

A Potential complications include: bad scars, infection, delayed healing, bleeding, reduction in nipple sensation, asymmetry, and fat necrosis.

## 🔁 Patient's perspective

Jenny is a 21-year-old university student. She is 5 ft 2 inches in height and weighs 8 stone. Following puberty at age 13, her breasts developed quickly and continued to grow for several years. She is now a double 'H' cup. Her large breasts caused her to give up her passion for dancing and she now avoids all forms of sport. She wears loose-fitting baggy clothes to disguise her shape. She feels unattractive and her confidence and self-esteem is low. Standing naked in front of a mirror, she burst into tears. She regarded her breasts as deformities and had often thought about the possibility of surgery and now decided to do something about it.

Jenny used the internet to research the procedure and to find a surgeon and found hundreds of sites with detailed information. She joined a chat room for women who had either had a breast reduction or were considering it. It was helpful to hear of real women's experiences and she was encouraged that most of them were delighted with the results of their surgery. Many women stressed the importance of finding a properly qualified surgeon with plenty of experience. By researching the sources of information on the internet, Jenny drew up a list of criteria for choosing a surgeon. This included:

- a fully trained and qualified plastic surgeon specializing in breast surgery

- reassurance that the consultation would be with the surgeon who would perform the procedure

- that she could see photographs of the results of surgery for women with similar breasts to her own

- being offered the opportunity to talk to one of the surgeon's previous patients

- confirming that she would receive seamless aftercare and follow-up

- information on the cost of surgery and, in particular, the financial implications of treatment for any complications or revisional procedures.

Jenny told her parents of her decision and that she would like to have surgery during the university holiday so she could recover in her own home
with the support of her family. She narrowed the search for a surgeon working in or around her area and arranged consultations with two of them.

At the first consultation, her mother accompanied her. Jenny was
delighted that the female surgeon encouraged her mother to sit in on the
consultation. She briefly summarized her experience and qualifications,
and Jenny found it reassuring to know that most of her time was devoted
to breast surgery and that she worked with a team reconstructing breasts
after cancer surgery.

The surgeon asked Jenny lots of questions about her general health and
past medical history, including any breast problems with women in Jenny's
family. She asked Jenny why she wanted surgery and encouraged her to
discuss the problems she had experienced as a result of her large breasts.

She then explained the procedure of breast reduction in detail, and listed
all the possible problems and complications. She emphasized the need to
accept scars and the possibility of interfering with nipple sensation. Jenny
was reassured to hear that breastfeeding was usually possible after surgery,
although she was also a little dismayed to learn that it was possible her
breasts might grow again with future pregnancy.

The surgeon examined her breasts and took several measurements. She
also took some photographs. Her weight and height were recorded. Jenny
was relieved to hear the surgeon confirm that she was a good candidate
for breast reduction. She was given an information booklet about the
surgery and its effects. The surgeon encouraged her to consider all the
issues raised and discuss them with friends and family. She also offered to
see Jenny again for a second consultation if she wanted to proceed, which
was offered free of charge.

In the car on the way home, Jenny told her mother that she had felt very
confident and comfortable with the surgeon, and that she did not want to
see anyone else. The following day, Jenny called the surgeon's secretary to
schedule a second consultation and enquire as to possible dates for surgery.

At the second consultation, Jenny was able to ask several questions, including practical aspects about recovery time, removal of stitches, and restrictions on physical activity. She learned that she would need to wear a support bra for a few weeks and would recover in plenty of time to return to university for the new term.

On the day of surgery, her surgeon and anaesthetist came to see her. The surgeon spent 20 minutes drawing on her breasts with a marking pen. When she had finished, she took more photographs. Jenny then signed the consent form. The anaesthetist reviewed her medical history and examined her heart and lungs with a stethoscope. She talked about medication for pain relief and that she would take a course of antibiotics for 10 days after surgery. Jenny could not believe that in a few hours she would finally have a new shape and be rid of the burden of her heavy pendulous breasts.

When she woke up in the recovery ward after her operation, Jenny was pleased to realize that she felt no pain at all. For the rest of the day she drifted in and out of sleep. She was vaguely aware of her surgeon and anaesthetist visiting her and reassuring her that the operation had gone as planned.

The following morning, she felt very well and enjoyed breakfast. Even though her breasts were partially hidden from view in a surgical bra, she was overjoyed. She could tell that she now had breasts that suited her size and shape. A nurse removed her drains (drainage tubes) and reviewed her postoperative instructions. After the pharmacy delivered her painkillers and antibiotics, her mother arrived to take her home.

The day after surgery, the practice nurse called her at home to check on her progress and confirm her follow-up appointment. Eight days later, Jenny returned to the surgeon's office and all her stitches were removed. Here, for the first time, she was able to see her new breasts. She barely registered the fading bruises or the neat scars and was thrilled with her new shape and size.

Six months later, Jenny saw her surgeon again. She felt like a different person, being able to wear whatever clothes she wanted, play badminton, swim, and run. She felt so much more confident. Her scars were beginning to fade and the redness had virtually gone. They were a small price to pay.

# Breast reduction for men

Breast tissue is present in men and women. At puberty, female sex hormones (oestrogen) stimulate breast development in girls. In some circumstances, breast tissue can develop in men, a condition known as 'gynaecomastia'. Gynaecomastia may develop during puberty. It can also occur as a result of weight gain, some medication and drugs (including steroids and marijuana), hormonal imbalance, liver disease, and rare inherited conditions such as Klinefelter syndrome. Advancing age and weight gain may predispose to fatty deposits in the breast area, so-called 'man boobs'.

Most men are embarrassed and distressed by this condition and are often highly motivated to seek a surgical correction.

## Assessment

Any consultation with a cosmetic surgeon should include a full medical history. This will determine if there is any underlying cause or condition that may result in breast development. Blood tests may also be performed to exclude any metabolic or hormonal imbalance. If any hormonal disturbance is suspected, referral to an endocrinologist may be appropriate.

Height and weight measurements are used to calculate the 'body mass index'. This is a useful guide to identifying and grading obesity. Lifestyle changes, including diet and exercise, will improve general health and reduce fat deposition in the chest area.

## Surgery

There are several different surgical options to treat gynaecomastia. The choice of operation depends on the type and severity of the condition.

Gynaecomastia can be broadly subdivided into three groups or 'grades'. These are:

*Grade 1:* localized distinct breast tissue, situated under the nipple area. There is no extra fat or loose skin. It is often seen in young men at or soon after puberty. Complete removal can be achieved through scars around the areola.

*Grade 2:* diffuse fatty excess of tissue with no distinct edges and little or no skin excess. It is usually suitable for treatment by liposuction through one or two small incisions.

*Grade 3:* diffuse excess of fatty tissue with excess skin. This may give the appearance of a female breast. Treatment of the most severe form of breast development with excess skin is difficult. Surgery will involve the presence of scars on the chest, similar to those produced by breast reduction in women.

#  Patient's perspective

When I was 16, I was tall and slim. During puberty, I noticed some swelling and tenderness around my nipples. The swelling carried on and I was horrified to realize that I had breasts. I enjoyed athletics and represented my school. Once, in the showers after training, another boy shouted for everyone to come and look at my 'tits'. Since then, I have given up sport and swimming. Even on holiday, I keep a baggy T-shirt on at all times.

I read an article in the paper about gynaecomastia. I was so excited as there was a story about someone just like me who had an operation. I explained to my parents that I wanted to have an operation. They were surprised at first as even they hadn't realized the problem and how upset I was. Once they understood, they were really great and agreed to support me and pay for the treatment.

Our general practitioner referred me to a breast surgeon who had a lot of experience with my condition. At the consultation, I was asked a lot of questions. The examination was a bit embarrassing as the surgeon checked my testicles were normal. He assured me they were! He explained that my problem was actually quite common and that many boys developed some breast swelling during puberty. Because mine were quite noticeable, he agreed that an operation was necessary. There would be scars but only around the edge of the darker nipple skin.

A month later, I went into hospital and had the op. They put me to sleep and I woke up with a tight-fitting garment like a vest with a zip up the front. I went home later on the same day. For a few days, my chest was sore and I took painkillers regularly.

A week after the op, I saw the surgeon and his nurse in the outpatient clinic at the hospital. The garment and the dressings were removed and some small stitches were taken out. When I looked in the mirror, I had some bruising on the skin but was delighted to see how flat my chest looked. I felt normal!

# 5

# Mastopexy

## → Key points

- Scars are an inevitable consequence of surgery to lift the breasts.

- Restoring fullness and projection of the breast may require the use of a breast implant as part of the procedure.

- Time, gravity, and subsequent pregnancy may cause recurrent drooping of the breast.

- Mastopexy can restore empty, droopy breasts to a more youthful, perkier, and fuller shape.

With age, gravity, weight loss, and breastfeeding, the breasts often lose their elasticity and volume. The skin and breast tissue may droop and sag and the areola enlarges. The perkiness and fullness of the youthful breast is lost. The degree of droopiness is variable. It may just involve a slight lowering of the nipple or the whole breast. A simple test is to stand with a pencil held under the breast crease (the so-called 'pencil test')—Does the pencil fall to the floor or is it held in place by the weight and position of a sagging or droopy breast? Droopiness (ptosis) can be graded by the degree of lowering of the nipple areola complex below the breast crease (Figure 5.1).

Surgery to restore the youthful shape and volume of the breast is called a mastopexy or 'breast lift'. Generally, the surgery is more complicated than straightforward breast enlargement and produces more scars. Mild to moderate cases can be performed with scars limited to around the areola. More significant ptosis correction will usually need a 'vertical' scar between the nipple and the breast base. Another scar may be required horizontally in the breast crease.

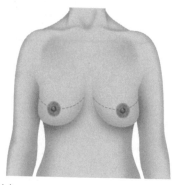
(a)

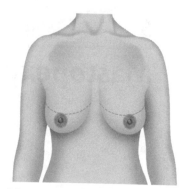
(b)

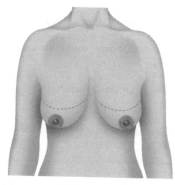
(c)

**Figure 5.1** (a–c) Three degrees of breast ptosis.

For droopy breasts that are empty with little volume, it is usual to combine a breast lift with an implant. This is known as 'augmentation mastopexy'. This operation is popular and can restore an attractive shape and size to the breast. However, there are well-recognized limitations and the risks and complications should be clearly explained.

## Assessment

As with any procedure, clients should be fit and healthy with no active medical problems—any history of breast cancer in the family should be declared. It is also important to have realistic expectations. Looking at photographs of results is a very useful way of appreciating the scars.

Your surgeon should assess the degree of ptosis (sag) and the need for an implant. The pattern of scars will be explained for the suggested procedure. If the breasts are large and droopy, a mastopexy may not need to include an implant.

## Surgical techniques and procedures

All breast-lift procedures involve lifting the nipple areola to the centre of the breast. They may also require tightening of the breast skin and repositioning of the breast tissue higher on the chest and may include the insertion of an implant at the same time. If the areola has stretched and enlarged, this is reduced as part of the procedure.

The scars may be confined to the perimeter of the nipple areolar complex for minor to moderate degrees of sag. These procedures are referred to as crescentic nipple elevation or the 'Benelli' technique. More significant procedures will add a scar running vertically down from the nipple to the base of the breast. These scar patterns are often referred to as the 'lollipop' or 'vertical scar'. The most extensive corrections produce an 'inverted T' scar, which runs around the nipple, down to the base of the breast and transversely in the breast crease (the inverted T scar). (See Figure 5.2 overleaf.)

## Complications

A procedure involving an implant carries the same risks as a straightforward augmentation. Mastopexy has specific potential problems including:

- longer scars

- nipple and skin numbness

- fat necrosis

- glandular 'drop out' where the nipple remains high but the breast drops lower on the chest wall

- variable nipple shape that may be more oval than round

- a more obviously 'implanted' look.

Fat necrosis occurs when breast tissue and fat loses its blood supply and results in hardening and lumpiness. In the first few weeks after surgery this may result in an oily discharge from the breast. In the longer term, the lumpiness may take up to 2 years to soften.

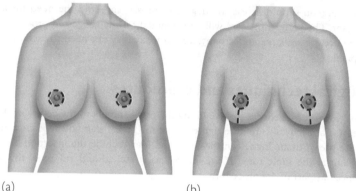

(a)  (b)

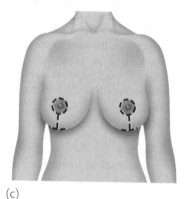

(c)

**Figure 5.2** Scars associated with mastopexy, including (a) periareolar, (b) short vertical scar, and (c) inverted 'T'.

Despite the best efforts of surgery, the breast tissue may continue to descend with time. This usually occurs under the nipple and may result in the nipple appearing to be situated high up on the breast. Recurrent droopiness can be minimized by wearing a bra but the relentless effect of gravity eventually prevails. Revision procedures can be performed if necessary.

Some reduction in nipple sensation can occur, although this is relatively rare.

When a droopy breast is associated with loss of breast tissue, an implant is almost always needed to fill the breast and restore projection. In these circumstances, there is little tissue to cover the implant and the breast may have a round appearance and be more obviously 'surgical'.

Despite the limitations of mastopexy and the scars, most women still prefer the results of surgery to a droopy, empty breast.

Immediately after surgery, the breasts will be shiny and swollen. It is important to understand that the shape of the breast will change in the first few months, becoming softer and more natural.

## 🛈 Patient's perspective

Joanne is 38 years old. She has three children aged 7, 4, and 2 and breast-fed all of them for several months. After her last pregnancy, her breasts were empty with loose skin. The areolae had become stretched and large and her nipples pointed downwards. She had lost all her pregnancy weight and exercised regularly. Despite being fit and toned, she was dismayed by the appearance of her breasts, which she thought looked like ' her grand-mother's. Her self-esteem and confidence were undermined and she avoided undressing in front of her husband and only engaged in sexual activity in darkness.

She read an article in a woman's lifestyle magazine, which featured breast-lift surgery and the experience of several women who had undergone the procedure. Joanne had a good relationship with her GP and asked her for advice and help in finding a reputable surgeon. Her GP knew of two local plastic surgeons with an interest in cosmetic breast surgery. She had previously referred other patients and had seen pleasing results of their work.

Joanne made an appointment to see one of the surgeons and attended a consultation with her husband. The consultation lasted for 50 minutes. Before examining Joanne, the surgeon took a full medical history and explained the nature, limitations, and potential complications of breast-lift surgery.

After the examination, the surgeon explained that Joanne would need to have a lift that involved scars around the nipple, down to the base of the breast and in the breast crease. She would also need a small breast implant to restore lost volume. He showed her photographs of the results of his work in other patients with similar breast shapes.

Joanne and her husband discussed all the issues raised in the consultation. She felt strongly motivated to proceed with surgery and that the benefits would outweigh the potential disadvantages.

After booking a date for surgery, Joanne saw the surgeon for a second consultation. She had a list of questions prepared after she had researched the operation on the internet, which her surgeon answered fully.

On the day of surgery, her surgeon prepared for the operation by making several measurements and markings on her breasts. The only one she remembered was the intended new position of her nipple in a higher position on the breast.

When Joanne came round after the operation, she experienced only mild discomfort. She slept reasonably well with the help of medication and painkillers. The following morning, a nurse removed the drains (clear plastic tubes) that the surgeon had placed during the procedure. The surgeon visited before she went home and gave her an information sheet with a list of do's and don't's and contact telephone numbers. The day after surgery, the surgeon's practice nurse phoned her at home to check all was well. She wore a support bra continuously for 10 days after the operation. Joanne returned to the surgeon's office where the nurse removed her stitches and saw her new breasts for the first time. She had been warned to expect that they would look swollen and full, 'as if you were breast feeding'. Although this was indeed the case, Joanne was delighted to see that her breasts were perky and the nipple was in a 'normal' position.

Six weeks after the operation, Joanne thought that most of the swelling had gone and her new breasts felt quite soft and natural. She was now back to normal activities, including working out in the gym. Three months later, she treated herself by buying new lingerie. She was pleased that the scars seemed to be healing well. She felt much more confident with her body.

# ❓ FAQ

Q1  Am I a suitable candidate for mastopexy?

A  If your breasts have sagged or drooped and appear empty with excess skin, a mastopexy could restore a more youthful appearance with better projection and fullness. It will also lift the breast and give a firmer, perkier appearance. Provided you accept the need for scars, have realistic expectations and good general health, a mastopexy can be a highly satisfying procedure.

Q2  I want to have more children. Should I have surgery now or wait until my family is complete?

A  Each pregnancy will result in swelling of the breast and stretching of the skin. Breast tissue may shrink (involute) to some degree after delivery. In general, it is probably wise to defer surgery if further pregnancies are planned.

Q3  I want a breast uplift, but have been told that I also need a breast implant. Is this really necessary?

A  Many women can have a mastopexy without the need for a breast implant. However, if the breast is very loose and empty, a mastopexy alone cannot restore volume. In these circumstances, an attractive breast shape may require an implant as well as a lift.

Q4  Where are the scars and are they permanent?

A  All mastopexy operations involve scars on the breasts. The pattern of scars depends on the degree of droopiness. Mild to moderate lifts can be performed with scars limited to the perimeter of the areola (the darker skin around the nipple). More significant correction may require a scar extending vertically downwards from the centre of the nipple towards the base of the breast (lollipop or vertical scar), and also a transverse scar in the crease of the breast (inverted 'T' or anchor pattern).

# 6

# Abdominoplasty

**➡ Key points**

◆ There are many different procedures available depending on individual circumstances.

◆ The operation may not be appropriate for patients who are overweight or have other medical problems.

◆ Abdominoplasty has the potential to cause serious and even life-threatening complications.

◆ Surgery should only be performed in a well-equipped hospital with highly trained staff.

A smooth, flat belly with a defined waist is an integral part of our perception of an attractive youthful body. Images of trim, muscular, bodies are everywhere, and used to market a variety of products from clothes to perfumes. Modern fashion trends have encouraged exposure of the belly and adornment with piercings.

Relatively few people are blessed with this aesthetic ideal, even in youth. The abdominal area is usually the first place affected by weight gain and an increase in waist size is almost inevitable with age. Fat deposition in the abdomen is different for men and women. Men tend to deposit fat internally in the abdominal cavity, whereas for women, fat is laid down in the subcutaneous layer.

Exercise and dieting are universally accepted as means of limiting and reducing fat and toning muscles. This is clearly desirable and has particular relevance for men as abdominal obesity is known to be a risk factor for heart disease.

Even with a healthy lifestyle, ageing results in loss of skin elasticity and a decrease in muscle tone, and an increased tendency for fat to accumulate.

However, the single, most significant factor responsible for irreversible changes to a youthful abdomen is pregnancy. During pregnancy, the skin and muscles of the abdominal wall are stretched to accommodate the growing baby. Fat may be deposited in and around the hips and thighs. After delivery, the skin may never quite be as smooth and tight as it was before pregnancy. Extra loose skin may remain and 'stretch marks' appear. The paired linear muscles, the rectus abdominis, may separate, allowing the belly to bulge. Fat deposits around the central abdomen are often notoriously difficult to shift. In addition to these anatomical changes, new mothers have little time for exercise. Caesarean section adds the further insult of muscle injury and a scar. The impact of pregnancy may vary from person to person and is often more severe with big babies or twins. The effects are usually more pronounced in older women. The changes frequently worsen with each subsequent pregnancy. So, after two or three pregnancies a woman may often be left with a permanent legacy that cannot be corrected by diet or exercise. She may have loose floppy skin with or without stretch marks, a thicker waist, and a permanent bulge. For many women, these changes can be profoundly depressing. In addition to restrictions on clothing such as swimwear and lingerie, the appearance may result in anxiety and depression with a lowering of confidence and self-esteem.

> ## 🛈 Patient's perspective
>
> The comments of one of my patients are typical:
>
> 'I look at myself naked in the bathroom mirror and feel so sad. My tummy looks disgusting, I feel so unattractive. I know my husband must be turned off. How could he not be? I never undress in front of him and only have sex with the lights off. I don't want to go on holiday this year. I couldn't go on a beach like this.'
>
> These feelings, and the knowledge that no amount of exercise or dieting will help, prompt many women to consider surgery.

## What is abdominoplasty?

Abdominoplasty or 'tummy tuck' includes a range of surgical procedures tailored to individual needs. The choice of procedure depends on an expert assessment of anatomy, weight, general health, and expectations. If the problem is only excess fat, abdominal liposuction may be used without the need for formal surgery (see Chapter 7). Liposuction may be used as part of formal abdominoplasty procedures.

Removal of excess skin and fat can be achieved with a 'mini abdominoplasty'. If the abdominal muscles need to be tightened, a 'full abdominoplasty' is required. Both these procedures involve scars in the lower abdominal crease, just above the pubic hair line . Another scar may be needed around the umbilicus (belly button).

Abdominoplasty can be very effective in improving the changes resulting from ageing and pregnancy. However, this is achieved with the trade-off of scars and accepting that the restoration of pre-pregnancy appearance may not be possible. In particular, stretch marks may be diminished and reduced but they cannot be removed.

In recent years, new techniques have been introduced to improve the aesthetic results. These have included procedures that enhance the waistline and modify the pattern of skin excision to avoid stretched scars. The most popular is the so-called 'high lateral tension' technique, developed by an American surgeon, Ted Lockwood.

## Suitable candidates for abdominoplasty

They should:

- not be obese

- have good general health

- have realistic expectations

- accept the scars and recovery period

- ideally have no plans for further pregnancies

- be non-smokers.

## Assessment and suitability

A consultation should include a thorough enquiry of your health status. Obesity, diabetes, history of thrombosis, and heart disease may increase the risk of serious complications. Examination should include a calculation of your body mass index or 'BMI', a measure of body fat determined by a calculation based on height and weight for adult males and females. It may overestimate fat in athletes with a large muscle mass and underestimate fat in the elderly and those with muscle wasting. It is not applicable for children. For most people, however, it is a useful guide to determine if you are overweight and to what degree. BMI categories:

◆ Underweight = <18.5

◆ Normal weight = 18.5–24.9

◆ Overweight = 25–29.9

◆ Obesity = 30 or greater.

To calculate your BMI, go to http://www.nhlbisupport.com/bmi or any similar site on the internet.

As a general rule, abdominoplasty should not be offered if your BMI is 25 or above. Instead, advice regarding diet and exercise is appropriate to lose weight and thus reduce the complications and increase the benefit of any surgery.

During pregnancy, the long paired muscles on either side of the midline (the rectus abdominis muscles) may be pushed to the side. After delivery, they may not come back to their original position, producing a bulge that may not respond to exercise or diet. The abdominal examination should assess muscle function and position.

It is also important to note any previous surgery and scars. Some scars may have an effect on the blood supply of the skin of the abdomen and be a potential reason for poor healing after abdominoplasty. Some bulges or 'hernias' may be present around the umbilicus (belly button) or groin area. They may be present since childhood but can develop with increasing weight, age, and after surgery or childbirth. If they are present, it may be possible and important to repair them at the same time as an abdominoplasty.

Anyone considering abdominoplasty should accept:

◆ the scars

◆ a minimum of 2 weeks recovery time

◆ some numbness of the lower abdominal skin

◆ the need for exercise and weight control after surgery

◆ the possible need for minor secondary surgery after 6 months.

# The operation

The procedure involves a general anaesthetic and an overnight stay in hospital.

All types of abdominoplasty result in a scar across the lower abdomen. This runs just above the pubic region in the same place as a caesarean section scar. It is longer than a caesarean scar and extends out towards the hips. A well designed scar should still be concealed by underwear or swimwear.

The tissues of the abdomen are separated from the underlying muscles. These muscles are often tightened before the excess skin is removed. The flap of excess skin and fat is drawn down to the lower incision and all excess skin is removed: a new hole is made in the skin to reveal the umbilicus (tummy button), which is stitched into its new position (Figure 6.1). Drainage tubes are almost always used and are usually removed the day after surgery.

An elasticated garment or binder is normally used to provide support and limit swelling for 10–14 days. During this time, physical activity will be limited and precludes driving a motor vehicle. Pain and discomfort often results from the muscle repair and may require painkilling medication for several days. Stitches are removed about 10 days after surgery. At this stage, improvement in the shape and contour of the abdomen is obvious. However, there will still be significant swelling of the tissues and improvement continues for up to 3 months. After 4–6 weeks, exercise may be gradually resumed. After muscle

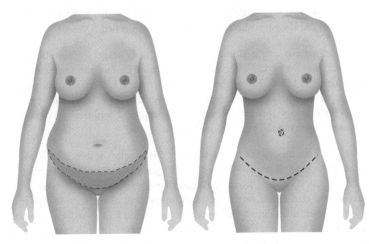

**Figure 6.1** Typical scars of abdominoplasty.

repair, a formal regimen of abdominal exercise is essential to regain tone and strength to maximize the benefit of surgery. Help from a physiotherapist or personal trainer is often useful.

A healthy diet is also essential to prevent weight gain.

## Complications

There are several well-recognized complications that may occur following surgery. These include:

- bleeding

- swelling and bruising

- seroma formation (this results from the accumulation of tissue fluid in the space between the muscles and the soft tissues; it may need to be drained off several times using a needle and syringe)

- red, raised scars

- numbness of the skin of the lower abdomen

- wound infections and delayed healing.

Rarely, more serious complications can occur. The risk of these is increased by obesity, diabetes, and a history of clotting disorders. Surgery should not be offered to patients with a BMI greater than 30 and judiciously if the BMI is higher than 25. Diabetes should be stable and controlled.

Any identified risk of developing blood clots after surgery (thromboembolic disease) should be carefully evaluated. It may require the use of medication to thin the blood during the perioperative period. Generally, all patients undergoing the procedure are treated with elasticated stockings and many are fitted with 'leggings' that provide regular inflation and compression to encourage blood flow from the veins in the legs.

If, despite these precautions, a blood clot does develop, it may often produce a swelling in the calf area of the leg. A venogram investigation will confirm if a clot is present. If it is, anticoagulation therapy will be started, which often dissolves the clot. If the clot detaches from the wall of the vein, it may travel to the arteries in the lungs and result in chest pain and shortness of breath. Again, in this situation, prompt treatment with blood-thinning medication is required to dissolve the clot.

Very rarely, complications can occur if the internal organs are damaged during the procedure. This can occur when a liposuction cannula has pierced the abdominal cavity and injured the bowel. When this occurs, it often results in high-profile media coverage, which understandably deters potential patients. Even if this unfortunate complication occurs, the symptoms should alert the surgeon to the possibility of internal damage. Prompt treatment, often with the help of an abdominal surgical colleague is usually effective in repairing any injury and allowing a full recovery.

Wound infections are usually minor, although they may delay healing in the incisions. Rarely, wound infections may be more serious if particular combinations of bacteria are present. In these situations, prompt expert treatment with specific antibiotics are needed to prevent tissue damage and the spread of the infection to the bloodstream, known as septicaemia. In theory, this complication can be life threatening.

It must be emphasized that these serious complications are extremely rare. However, in a published scientific review of a large number of patients, the incidence of all complications, however minor, was documented at 24%!

For a particular group of patients, the desire for surgery may arise as a result of the effects on the body of massive weight loss. Often, this is a result of surgical procedures designed for this purpose. These operations include gastric bypass or gastric banding, which limit food intake and result in weight loss. The procedures may be so effective that massive reduction in weight can result. This surgery is often referred to as 'bariatric' surgery. Bariatric patients are then often confronted with the consequences of their dramatic weight loss. They are frequently left with large folds of excess skin evident in many areas, including the face, neck, arms, breasts, abdomen, thighs, and buttocks.

In the abdominal area, they usually require an abdominoplasty procedure but it may need to be more extensive than the conventional operation. The need to remove large amounts of skin circumferentially has stimulated specific surgical solutions. The operation is frequently referred to as a 'body lift'. This is a much more extensive procedure than a traditional abdominoplasty. It takes more time and the scars are more extensive, encircling the entire torso. The operation may also incorporate a buttock and thigh lift at the same time. Surgeons offering this treatment usually have extra training and expertise and may be 'specialists' in this field. They will, in addition to body lifts, perform arm and thigh reductions and breast reduction and reshaping when appropriate.

## Thigh lift

After weight loss or with loss of skin tone, the skin and soft tissue of the inner thighs may become loose or lax. When there is an excess of skin, this can be removed and tightened by a procedure known as a thigh lift. This involves incisions that run around the tops of the thighs into the buttock crease. These wounds are uncomfortable during the recovery period and limit full activity for 3 or 4 weeks.

## Arm lift

Loose skin under the arms can be very distressing and restrict the choice of clothing. When very severe, removal of the excess skin can be performed. Arm-lift surgery, however, is unpopular with most surgeons as the scars produced may be unsightly and still need to be covered.

# Conclusions

For the mainstream patient with excess abdominal skin and fat, an abdominoplasty can produce an excellent improvement in the shape and contour of the tummy. This can be extremely rewarding and improve self-esteem and confidence. Many women report their delight at being 'given back their body'. They are delighted to be able to wear fashionable clothes and often experience a return of their sexual confidence. Most consider the scar a small price to pay.

# ❓ FAQ

Q1  Is an abdominoplasty an option for me?

A  If you are in good general health and not significantly overweight, an abdominoplasty can be highly effective in improving the changes that often result from pregnancies, weight loss, and the ageing process. These changes include permanent folds of excess skin, excess abdominal fat that doesn't respond to diet or exercise and bulging of the tummy as a result of muscle laxity.

Q2  What does the operation involve?

A  Abdominoplasty or 'tummy tuck' may refer to several different operations. These may vary from a limited removal of excess skin (a mini tummy tuck) to a more extensive procedure requiring the simultaneous removal of skin and fat, liposuction and repair of the abdominal muscles. There are several designs of skin excision and scar patterns.

Q3  Who isn't a good candidate for this surgery?

A  Poor results and higher complication rates are likely in patients who are significantly overweight. Surgeons quantify this by calculating the 'body mass index' or BMI for each candidate. The calculation is performed with each person's height and weight. In general, normal body weight gives a reading of less than 25. A person is overweight if the BMI is between 25 and 30. A figure above 30 is indicative of obesity. Many surgeons will decline to operate on anyone with a BMI greater than 25 and almost all would exclude anyone with a BMI greater than 30.

In addition, surgery may be inappropriate for patients with unstable diabetes, high blood pressure, ischaemic heart disease, and a history of clotting disorders. The latter may predispose a potential patient to develop blood clots in the leg and pelvic veins after surgery. If this occurs, it may lead to death if the clots detach and lodge in the lungs. Finally, surgery should only be offered to patients who are psychologically stable and accept the limitations and complications of surgery.

Q4  What are the complications that can occur after surgery?

A  Like all surgical procedures, bleeding and infection may occur. These are rare and can normally be dealt with successfully. Very rarely, an unusual aggressive infection may result in tissue death and a generalized infection in the whole body called septicaemia. If severe, this may even be life threatening.

A more common problem is the development of a 'seroma'. This occurs when tissue fluid accumulates between the muscle layer and the skin and fat layer of the abdomen. Usually, this is self-limiting and the tissue fluid resorbs, although it may require surgical drainage with a needle on several occasions.

Some people may have a tendency to form red, raised, and thick scars, which may be unsightly or even painful. There are several methods of improving scars but this may take time and the improvement can be variable.

Rarely, a complication may result from a surgical error. Abdominoplasty is often performed with liposuction. If the liposuction cannula (a metal tube) penetrates the abdominal cavity, it can cause damage to the internal abdominal organs, including the bowel, liver, or spleen. It is essential that this complication is promptly recognized and treated to avoid serious illness and even death. Fortunately, this problem is extremely rare.

Q5 How long before I can return to work?

A Even after most types of full abdominoplasty, return to work is usual after 2 weeks. However, you may still not be capable of unrestricted physical activity and you may still need to wear an abdominal support garment.

Q6 Will the operation remove my stretch marks?

A Stretch marks are the silvery lines that often arrive after a pregnancy or gain in weight. They represent damage to the collagen fibres in the skin and can be thought of a 'fracture' or 'tear' within the skin. Despite claims to the contrary, there is no effective treatment to remove stretch marks. During abdominoplasty, some stretch marks will be lost with the extra skin that is removed but in the skin that remains they will still be present.

## *i* Patient's perspective

Susan is 38 years old and has three children aged 7, 5, and 3. Her third child was delivered by Caesarian section. Following the birth of the first two children, Sue was pleased that her tummy had only a few stretch marks and returned pretty much to normal. However, after the third pregnancy, she was not so lucky. A year after delivery, she had lost almost all the weight gained during pregnancy and had worked really hard in the gym on her tummy muscles. Despite all her efforts, Sue was dismayed to find that she still had a floppy fold of extra skin and a permanent 'bulge' that was impossible to hide. She was shocked and upset when a friend asked her if she was pregnant again. She was depressed when she looked at her tummy in the mirror. Her negative feelings about her body eroded her confidence. She avoided intimacy with her husband. She felt intimidated by images of flat youthful abdomens in magazines and switched off the television whenever they appeared.

Sue realized that no amount of diet and exercise would reverse the changes resulting from childbirth. She refused to accept that nothing could be done to improve her appearance and had no hesitation in exploring the option of cosmetic surgery. She consulted her general practitioner, a woman approximately her own age. To her surprise and delight, her GP was not only sympathetic but revealed that she had herself undergone an abdominoplasty for much the same problems. With first-hand experience, she confirmed that Sue was an appropriate candidate and referred her to the same plastic surgeon who performed her own operation.

Sue wanted her husband to be involved in her decision to consider surgery and was pleased to find that the surgeon positively encouraged them both to attend the consultation. The surgeon began the consultation by asking a lot of questions about Sue's general health and medical history. This included details of her pregnancies, previous operations and anaesthetics; her height, weight, and blood pressure were all measured.

The examination of her abdomen included an assessment of the strength of her muscles and the type of scars that had resulted from her caesarian section. Photographs were taken in the standing position. After the examination, the surgeon confirmed that Sue would be a good candidate for an abdominoplasty or 'tummy tuck'. He explained that this would involve tightening the muscles and removing the excess skin. The benefits of the operation in tightening and flattening the tummy were only possible if Sue was prepared to accept some scars. These would be longer than her caesarian scar and may take several months to fade. Although they would not be visible when wearing lingerie or swimwear, they might always be visible when naked. The surgeon showed them several photographs of his previous patients with typical examples of the results and the scars. He also warned Sue that her lower abdomen might be numb for a year or two and that stretch marks could not be completely removed.

Regarding the operation, the surgeon emphasized that Sue would need to stay in hospital for at least one night and possibly two. She would have drainage tubes for a few days and would need to wear an abdominal support garment for several weeks. With three young children at home, he encouraged her and her husband to arrange for extra help for a week or so as physical activity would be restricted. The school run had to be covered as driving is not possible for 10–14 days!

After the consultation, Sue and her husband discussed all the issues involved in the option of surgery. Sue felt strongly motivated to have the operation. She was prepared to accept the discomfort and recovery time and much preferred the inevitable scars if it meant a flatter belly.

Having decided to go ahead, Sue and her husband scheduled a date for surgery. They arranged for Sue's mother to stay with them for a week after the operation to help with the children.

Sue had been given an information pack by the surgeon, which included advice and details of the preparation, surgery, and recovery process. She saw the surgeon again, a week before the operation to ask some final questions and have a blood test requested by the anaesthetist.

On the day of surgery, Sue arrived at the hospital at 7.30 a.m. After being admitted by the ward nurse, she saw the surgeon and signed the consent form and met the anaesthetist. She elected to have a 'premed', which made her feel relaxed and sleepy before being taken to theatre. Her next memory was waking up back in her room. She was aware of some discomfort in her abdomen but no real pain. A catheter had been placed in her bladder, which meant she didn't have to get up to pass urine. She had regular pain medication and dozed for most of the day and night.

The following day, she saw the surgeon and the anaesthetist again. The catheter was removed and she was encouraged to get up and walk along the ward corridor several times. She had arranged to stay for two nights. After another good nights sleep, the nurse removed her drains and changed her dressings.

She was given her medications, which included pain killers and antibiotics, and also received an instruction sheet with a list of do's and don't's and contact telephone numbers for the surgeons office and hospital staff. Back at home, Sue was grateful that they had arranged for some help with the children as she felt quite tired out after taking the recommended two short walks!

By the fourth postoperative day, she felt much stronger and much more active although she still felt exhausted at the end of the day and slept soundly for 10 hours. A week after surgery, her normal energy had returned and she was looking forward to being able to resume driving. Ten days after the op she attended an appointment with the surgeon and his nurse who removed the dressings and stitches. For the first time, she was able to look at her abdomen. She was delighted to see that her belly was flat and that all the folds of excess skin were gone. She didn't mind the scar, which looked very neat and was placed in a natural line just above the pubic hair. It was obvious that the tissues were a little puffy and swollen but she had been warned to expect that and knew it would return to normal after several weeks.

Six weeks after the operation, Sue had completely recovered and started exercising in the gym. She explained the operation to her personal trainer and they organized a schedule of abdominal exercises to improve muscle tone and strength. Although the scar was a little red, she was thrilled with her new shape and felt that her confidence was restored.

Six months later, she visited her surgeon for the final appointment. The scars had begun to fade and the results of the surgery and her abdominal workouts had been dramatic. Sue regained a toned flat tummy and her confidence. There are no regrets regarding her decision to undergo surgery. She asked her surgeon for a copy of the photograph taken before the operation. Once in a while, she takes it out and looks at it. The image of her body after childbirth makes her shudder. It seems to belong to someone else!

# 7

# Liposuction

## Key points

♦ Liposuction is the most popular procedure in cosmetic surgery.

♦ It is a procedure that improves body shape and contours, but is not a means of weight loss.

♦ The best results are achieved in patients under the age of 40 with good skin and muscle tone.

Liposuction, lipoplasty, liposculpture, and body contouring are all terms used to describe a surgical procedure using a cannula attached to a vacuum suction device to remove fat from various areas of the body.

Liposuction is the most popular of all cosmetic procedures worldwide. The technique was pioneered by a French surgeon, Yves-Gerard Illouez in 1977. He developed cannulae with blunt tips that allowed fat to be removed with minimal damage to the surrounding tissues. Since then, many modifications and improvements have taken place, and advances in technology have refined the surgical instruments and expanded the means by which the fat is removed. Liposuction can be removed using laser and ultrasound as an energy form to break up the fat to be suctioned. There are new technologies emerging that offer the prospect of dissolving fat without surgery, which include transcutaneous ultrasound and injections. At the moment their safety and effectiveness remains to be determined.

An American surgeon, Peter Fodor, and a dermatologist, Jeffrey Klein, introduced the practice of introducing a solution of fluids into the tissues before aspirating the fat. This reduces bleeding, swelling and recovery time. This method is now routine although there are variations in the composition and volume of fluid used. These procedures are often referred to as the 'wet' 'super wet', or 'tumescent' techniques. Ultrasound, laser, and power-assisted suction devices are examples of more recent attempts to refine and improve the results.

The idea of a simple procedure to remove unwanted fat has obvious appeal and the popularity of liposuction is understandable. However, achieving a good result depends on many factors, including patient selection.

Liposuction is not an operation for losing weight. It has virtually no place for the treatment of obesity. Rather, it should be viewed as an effective method of removing specific areas of fat that are resistant to a healthy lifestyle, diet, and exercise. The areas of fat suitable for liposuction include the abdomen, flanks, hips, thighs, and inner knees. Other less common areas may include the breasts and under the chin.

For women, the pattern of fat deposition in certain areas can be genetic and influenced by hormones and ageing. Fat in the hip and thigh area may result in a 'pear'-shaped or 'gynoid' body shape. This may be evident even in youth. (See Figure 7.1.)

The pattern of fat deposition in men is different and almost always affects the abdomen (android body shape). Frequently, men may store fat inside the abdomen around the abdominal organs, which is not removable. The chest area may also be affected and deposits in the pectoral area can result in 'man boobs'. Swelling in the breast area in men can be genetic and may be caused by a variety of medications (see Chapter 4).

Although liposuction is perceived as a minor and minimally invasive technique, it is still a surgical procedure. Suitability may depend on many factors. These include:

- good general health

- realistic expectations

- a localized problem area of fat

- age

- skin tone or elasticity.

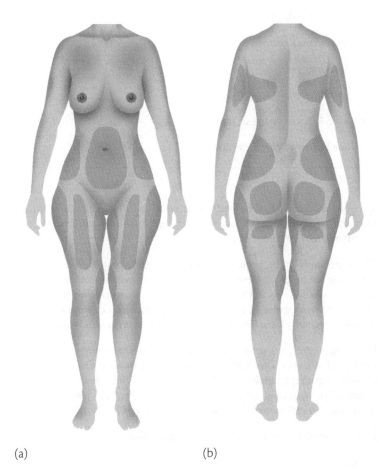

(a)　　　　　　　　　　　　　　　　　(b)

**Figure 7.1** (a,b) Body shape showing fat deposition in the hip and thigh area (gynoid).

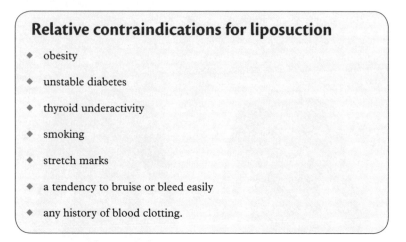

## Relative contraindications for liposuction

- obesity

- unstable diabetes

- thyroid underactivity

- smoking

- stretch marks

- a tendency to bruise or bleed easily

- any history of blood clotting.

The operation can often be performed under local anaesthesia or sedation ('twilight' anaesthesia). If a large amount of fat is to be removed, a general anaesthetic may be a better option.

There are limits to the amount of fat that can be removed in one procedure. Removing too much fat (several litres) may result in dangerous imbalances in the bodies fluids. Also, if a very large amount of fat is removed from an area, the skin in this area may be loose. Although excess skin can contract with time (as after pregnancy), the ability to do this depends on age and skin tone.

Following surgery, it is almost always necessary to wear a surgical support garment for 2–4 weeks. This limits swelling, reduces discomfort, and encourages the skin to re-drape tightly around the treated area. Scars from liposuction are minimal. The cannula is introduced into the tissues through a few small incisions measuring 3–4 millimetres. These are discreetly placed and usually heal well.

Excellent areas for treatment by liposuction include:

- hips

- thighs

- abdomen

- inner knees

- flanks ('love handles')

◆ chin

◆ back of the neck (can accumulate excess fat as the result of treatment for HIV—this so-called 'buffalo hump' can be treated very effectively with liposuction).

Difficult areas include:

◆ calves

◆ back

◆ arms

◆ face.

For the right patient, the results can be dramatic. In the hip and thigh area, surgery may restore the waistline, streamline hips, and restore an aesthetic line to the thighs. It has often been referred to as 'surgery of the silhouette'.

## Complications

Among the complications are:

◆ bleeding

◆ infection

◆ scars

◆ contour irregularities

◆ lumpiness

◆ extra skin looseness

◆ fat necrosis.

### 𝑖 Patient's perspective

Vicky is a 24-year-old postgraduate art student. She is 5 ft 6 inches tall and weighs 9 stone 4 lbs. She enjoys sport and exercises regularly. She has always been conscious of her heavy hips and thighs. No amount of diet or exercise helped. In fact, she noticed that weight loss made her more aware of the problem as her breasts and upper body would be smaller and thinner, but her hips and thighs stayed the same. Looking at her body in a mirror, she felt that the lower half of her body did not match the upper half. This had practical problems. Being a size 8 in one part of her body and a size 12 in the other half made it difficult to find clothes that fitted. She avoided close-fitting dresses and shorts.

For a long time, Vicky had been aware that liposuction might be an option. She read articles in magazines and on the internet. From these, she became convinced it might help. She found a site with photographs of results in girls with a similar body shape to hers.

As a student, she had little money and a bank loan. She found several adverts for cosmetic surgery that offered to arrange interest free loans to pay for the surgery. She rang their advice lines and spoke to a cosmetic surgery counsellor, who was very enthusiastic about the operation. She even volunteered that she had had liposuction herself! The counsellor arranged an appointment to see Vicky, which was free of charge. Vicky was surprised to find that the consultation was in a residential house. The counsellor was very chatty and friendly. She examined Vicky and assured her that liposuction would make a huge difference. She reassured her that the surgeons at the clinic were very good and 'never had any problems'. Vicky was surprised to find that she would not meet the surgeon until the day of her admission to hospital.

She was also given a telephone number for the finance company that could arrange her loan. The counsellor also said that if Vicky booked there and then with a small deposit, she would be given a 10 per cent discount on the fees. Vicky felt a little pressurized by the inducements to commit on the spot and decided to think about it. She was uneasy that she could not meet the surgeon who would be operating on her before the day of surgery. She did ring the finance company and was pleased that they thought she would qualify for a loan.

Vicky had also seen a website listing all the surgeons belonging to a professional association of plastic surgeons. These were mainly Consultants in Plastic Surgery in NHS hospitals. Several of these declared an interest in cosmetic surgery and liposuction. Although the consultation fee was £150, Vicky arranged to see one of these surgeons.

The consultation took place in an outpatient suite in a private hospital. Vicky met with the surgeon who would be performing her operation. He took a detailed medical history and she was weighed and her height was recorded. She was also photographed. The surgeon explained that she would be a good candidate for liposuction and showed her photographs of the results of some of his other patients with similar body shapes. He explained the procedure and the postoperative care. She learned that she would have to wear a special support garment for 4 weeks after surgery to limit the swelling and bruising and that the final result would be seen after a few months. She was also introduced to the practice nurse and given an information pack with details of the procedure. Vicky felt much more confident with the approach of this surgeon. She was reassured to know that the surgeon and his nurse would be in charge of her care throughout her treatment.

Four weeks later, Vicky had her surgery and was very pleased with the results.

## ❓ FAQ

**Q1** I wanted to have fat removed from my back area but my surgeon refused as he said it wouldn't work. Is he right?

**A** Some areas respond better to liposuction than others. Most surgeons feel that the results of surgery for 'back fat' are disappointing. Sometimes, surgery can help to tighten the skin in this area as the scar produced under the surface contracts after surgery. This principle is often effective under the chin, but is less rewarding on the back.

**Q2** Is it true that the skin can be lumpy and uneven after liposuction?

**A** There is a risk of some unevenness or irregularity of the skin following surgery. This is usually minor and can often be smoothed out with a minor secondary procedure. More widespread lumpiness can occur if too much fat is removed from the area directly under the skin. The problem is also more common after the age of 50 and following removal of very large amounts of fat.

**Q3** Can liposuction improve cellulite?

**A** Cellulite is the appearance of dimpling in the skin caused by pockets of fat bulging between strands of fibrous tissue in the tissues underneath the skin. Liposuction is usually not very effective as a treatment.

Although claims are made for many non-surgical modalities, there is still no consistently reliable method of removing cellulite.

Q4 Can I have liposuction under local anaesthetic?

A Many liposuction procedures can be preformed under local anaesthetic. Larger procedures can also be performed under sedation or 'twilight' anaesthesia. If the procedure involves treatment of several areas, a general anaesthetic may be preferred. The option of general anaesthetic is more common in the UK than in the USA for several reasons including culture and cost. You should be offered the opportunity to discuss the various anaesthetic options with your surgeon and anaesthetist.

Q5 What is 'smart' liposuction?

A This term is seductive, if not very descriptive. Essentially, this procedure uses a cannula to direct laser energy at fat cells. Instead of suctioning or aspirating the fat out of the body, the technique relies on the disrupted fast cells being removed by the bodies own lymphovascular system. The technique has not yet demonstrated reliable long-term results and there are some potential complications from loading the body with globules of fat. Technologies continue to evolve and offer new possibilities for fat removal without surgery. These include the use of ultrasound energy to dissolve fat and injections of 'fat dissolving' enzymes. Neither of these procedures are currently licensed for use in the UK.

Q6 I have heard the operation can cause a lot of bruising. Is there any way of reducing this?

A Almost all liposuction surgery can and does result in some bruising. To avoid this, it is important to avoid taking an aspirin-containing medication or anti-inflammatory medication such as ibuprofen for 2 weeks before surgery. Many surgeons advocate the use of 'arnica', a herbal preparation that seems to be effective in minimizing bruising. After surgery, the use of a close-fitting garment is usually recommended. This has the advantage of minimizing swelling and bruising. If you know you bruise or bleed easily, it is likely you will experience more bruising after surgery. Sometimes, your surgeon may perform a blood test to check your blood clotting is normal.

# 8

# Facelift surgery

> ### ➔ Key points
>
> ◆ Facelift surgery is highly effective in reversing many features of the ageing face.
>
> ◆ Heavy smokers are not suitable for facelift surgery.
>
> ◆ To achieve a natural result, surgery to the eye and brow area may also be required.

The term 'facelift' is perhaps the most commonly used word associated with cosmetic surgery. It has entered the language to the degree that it is widely applied to describe restoration or rejuvenation of everything from buildings to institutions. Paradoxically, its meaning in cosmetic surgery is frequently poorly understood and used inappropriately.

## Features of the ageing face

The signs of ageing are universal. Loss of skin elasticity, thinning of the skin and loss of collagen and soft tissues result in folds and wrinkles. The effect of gravity results in the formation of jowls, loose folds of skin in the neck, loss of fullness in the cheekbone area, and deepening of the nose to mouth lines known as the nasolabial folds. The ageing face also loses volume of soft tissues, which results in a gaunt appearance. This can be likened to the effect of letting air out of a balloon. (See Figure 8.1.)

These changes obscure the features of a youthful face. The smooth jaw line is lost and the face appears longer. This is the basis for comments such as 'why the long face' or looking 'down in the mouth'. For women in particular, jowls result in a loss of an oval shape to the face. Loose neck skin and the

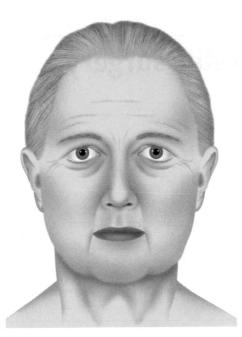

**Figure 8.1** Ageing face showing jowls, lax neck, and heavy nasolabial lines.

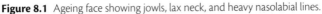

accumulation of fat under the chin reduce the youthful sharp angle between the chin and the neck.

Ageing in the face may be greatly accelerated by lifestyle and environmental influences, such as smoking, excess sun exposure, weight changes, pollution, and stress. The overall impact of ageing may result in a perception that the face looks stern or even angry. This is confirmed by comments from friends, family, and colleagues, like 'You look tired', 'Don't worry, it may never happen', 'Are you upset?'. These changes can also have practical consequences. It becomes more difficult to apply makeup, and loose neck skin often restricts choices of clothes and jewellery.

The social and psychological impact of ageing can be profound. Modern society places great emphasis on youth and attractiveness, which is associated with energy and success. In the workplace, an ageing appearance may generate anxiety about exclusion, ability, and promotion prospects. Socially, ageing may result in a loss of confidence and self-esteem. The loss of youthful features is also associated with sexual 'invisibility'. It has become much more difficult to 'grow old gracefully'.

Once physical changes have occurred, they will be permanent and will only increase with time. In modern society, many people in middle age are physically strong and healthy. They are often at the height of their careers. They will lament that they are young in mind, body, and spirit but are judged by their face, which is 'older than they are or feel'. They may be recently divorced or bereaved and considering new relationships, or are concerned that their face compromises their professional, social, and sexual potential.

These are some of the issues that may motivate people to consider the option of surgery.

## What is a facelift

What, then, is a facelift? The classical surgical procedure should probably be renamed a 'lower' facelift or 'neck lift'. This is because it does not address the features of ageing in the middle and upper parts of the face, including the area around the eyes and the forehead. These areas are improved by additional procedures such as blepharoplasty and brow lifts (see Chapter 10).

The classical 'facelift' can be very effective in reversing the effects of ageing in the neck and lower part of the face. These include:

◆ laxity or loosening of the tissues in the neck

◆ the development of 'jowls', with the loss of a clean jaw line

◆ deepening of the lines or folds of skin from the side of the nose running down to the corners of the mouth.

These signs of ageing are universal and arise as a result of the effects of gravity and the laxity of tissues that lose their elasticity with age. People with a history of excessive sun exposure may develop an inelastic leathery skin with many lines. This pattern of ageing is less responsive to facelift surgery.

Historically, surgical procedures to correct these changes were directed at lifting and tightening the skin. Although they were relatively successful, the results were often short lived and less than natural. Over the last 15–20 years, a better understanding of the process of facial ageing and advances in surgical techniques has produced a plethora of options for facial rejuvenation. The major types of facelifts include the following.

## Skin lift

This operation is now rarely performed. Although it can produce good results, the effects are often short lived. Removing too much skin can result in a taut 'operated' look.

## SMAS lift

Most modern procedures include tightening of the tissues under the skin including the muscles and fat, often referred to as the SMAS (subcutaneous musculoaponeurotic system). Traditional SMAS procedures have been modified to include the 'extended SMAS lift', the SMAS-ectomy, and the more conservative SMAS plication.

Facelift procedures that include tightening the SMAS are currently the most frequently performed, most reliable and effective methods of rejuvenating the ageing face.

## Deep plane and subperiosteal lift

These procedures lift all the facial tissues from the underlying bones of the face. They can deliver dramatic results but may result in a change in facial appearance. Recovery can be longer.

## Volumetric facelift

When the face is thin and gaunt, a standard facelift may be less effective and result in a tight, stretched look. A new approach in this situation is the 'volumetric' facelift. This procedure concentrates on restoring fullness to the face by injecting the patient's own fat into the face. The fat is taken from the abdomen or inside of the knees. It is then prepared for injection by removing excess oil and fluid. Using small needles and syringes, the fat is injected into the cheeks, chin, and lips. It can be used, with caution, around the eyes.

## MACS lift, soft lift, and thread lift

Recently, there has been a trend towards more minimal surgery with reduction in scars and the use of simple internal stitches, which include the so-called 'short scar', 'soft lift', and 'thread lift'. The effectiveness of these more minor operations is yet to be proven and there is concern that the results may be short lived.

# Assessment

Suitability for surgery depends on a number of factors that must be assessed by your surgeon. Anyone considering facelift surgery should be:

◆  medically fit

◆  tobacco free

◆  psychologically stable

◆  have clear goals and realistic expectations

◆  be prepared for some 'downtime'.

The decision as to which type of procedure is performed depends on an expert assessment of each persons needs. Factors influencing the choice include:

◆  the quality and thickness of the skin

◆  the degree of sun damage

◆  the amount of fat in the face

◆  the extent of skin laxity (looseness)

◆  the degree of jowling and neck laxity.

A facelift, as explained, is specifically targeted at the lower face and neck. In order to achieve a balanced natural rejuvenation of the whole face, it may be desirable to incorporate other procedures at the same time. These include brow lift, blepharoplasty, and fat transfer.

Prior to surgery, your general health should be assessed. Particular attention is paid to heart and lung problems, including high blood pressure, medication, allergies, and bleeding tendencies. Prior to surgery, some basic medical investigations may be performed, including blood tests, an ECG (electrocardiogram), and occasionally a chest X-ray. Facelift surgery is not advisable in heavy smokers as the risk of bleeding and poor healing is increased. Your surgeon may be able to offer help and support in giving up smoking.

Examination of the face will assess the degree of sun damage to the skin, the effects of gravity, the amount of fat and soft tissue in the face (facelift is more difficult with a thin face), the extent of bone loss (following loss of teeth), and the shape of the face. The technique used for a full face with good skin will be different for a thin face with leathery lined wrinkles. A tendency to 'yo-yo' in weight gain and weight loss may decrease the benefits of surgery.

After a thorough assessment of suitability, a surgeon may propose a surgical plan with clearly defined goals. The recovery period and potential complications should be clearly discussed.

# The procedure

A facelift is a surgical procedure. It is usually performed under general anaesthetic in a hospital environment with an overnight stay, although it is possible to have the procedure under local anaesthesia or sedation (so-called ' twilight' anaesthesia).

Often, a solution of anaesthetic and adrenaline is injected into the face to reduce bleeding and swelling. After the skin of the face has been elevated, the underlying muscles are tightened by various techniques. Extra skin is then removed and the wounds closed. Drains are usually placed and removed the following day. The operation usually takes between 2 and 3 hours.

## Postoperative care

The face may be dressed with a bandage or compressive dressing, which is normally removed the following day. Some swelling and bruising is inevitable giving a shiny, swollen effect that resolves after a week or two. Stitches are generally removed between the fifth and tenth postoperative day. Painkillers and antibiotics are often prescribed for 10 days or so.

For the first 12–24 hours after the operation, a head dressing or bandage is often used. The patient is nursed in a sitting position and may be gently sedated. The day after surgery, the dressings and drains are removed and the hair is washed. Most patients are then discharged from hospital. Specific information on postoperative care is provided to optimize a quick recovery During this time, patients are encouraged to sleep in a semi-upright position using several pillows As with all surgery there is a recovery period (downtime), which will restrict work, social, and sporting activity for a minimum of 2 weeks.

The vast majority of facelift procedures produce a scar that runs in front of and behind the ear (Figure 8.2). The scars are designed to follow natural skin creases and usually heal very well. They should be discrete enough to be invisible in social interactions; however, they may not escape the attention of your hairdresser. For the first few months after surgery they may be a little red

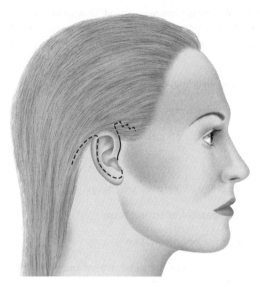

**Figure 8.2** Face showing facelift scars.

and raised and may require concealment with makeup. Usually, scar maturation can be assisted with the use of specific topical gels containing silicone. Very occasionally, a thicker scar may occur that can be treated by local steroid injections.

For men considering facelift, there are specific issues regarding the scar. Short hair limits the options for hiding the scars in the first few months after surgery. Moving the hair-bearing or beard areas of the skin may necessitate shaving behind the ear and around the front of the ear. It is possible to depilate these areas with electrolysis or with a laser.

The scar behind the ear may cause a 'step' in the hairline and wearing the hair up may be problematic. Occasionally a wide scar in this area can be very effectively concealed by hair transplants or grafts. Anxiety about scars has attracted interest in a number of techniques, which can be carried out with shorter scars. These include options that have no scar behind the ear, the so-called 'short scar' facelift. Another variant of the facelift limits scars to within the mouth and the scalp in the temporal region. These operations are often called 'endoscopic' facelifts as some of the surgery can be done using a camera through small incisions or cuts.

As with all surgery, there is a recovery period (downtime) that will restrict work, social, and sporting activity for a minimum of 2 weeks. Specific information on postoperative care is provided to optimize a quick recovery. Patients should avoid:

- lifting, straining, bending, or coughing

- any form of sexual activity

- excessive use of mobile phones.

They should:

- sleep on three pillows for a week after surgery

- be in a warm, tobacco-free environment

- take all their prescribed medication

- avoid taking aspirin or non-steroidal anti-inflammatory painkillers such as ibuprofen (Nurofen or Brufen).

Minimizing bruising in the immediate postoperative period usually results in a rapid and uncomplicated recovery. A degree of swelling and bruising is usual and may vary between individuals. It is normal for the cheeks to be numb for up to 3 months after surgery. Stitches are removed between 5 and 10 days after surgery. Most patients will need 2–3 weeks recovery before being socially presentable and able to return to work. Exercise and sexual activity should be avoided for 4–6 weeks after surgery. The healing process continues for a month or so and the final result is often at its best after 3 months.

A good result should be natural with no obvious signs of surgery. Patients usually report that friends and colleagues say they look 'well'. Frequently they will be asked if they have lost weight, had their hair done, or changed their makeup. It should not be evident that they have had 'work done'.

## How long does it last?

A facelift may turn back the clock but the ageing process continues. Following surgery, you will always look younger than you would have done. Most patients are content with one operation and it is a fallacy that 'once you have done it once you have to go back'. However, some patients do undergo repeat procedures after a period of 8–10 years, if physical changes recur.

# Complications

The commonest complication of a facelift is bleeding. This is rare and occurs in about 2–3% of cases; it usually develops in the first 12 hours after surgery and presents as a swelling on the side of the face. This is called a 'haematoma'. Prompt treatment is essential as if untreated it can lead to problems with healing and recovery. Usually, a haematoma necessitates a return to the operating theatre to remove the blood clot and stop the bleeding. Identified risk factors for haematoma include:

◆ smokers

◆ men

◆ high blood pressure

◆ medication such as aspirin, ibuprofen (Nurofen or Brufen), and other blood thinners

◆ operations involving surgery under the chin area—these may raise the pressure in the veins of the neck and face, leading to bleeding.

Nerve damage is often cited as an alarming potential complication of facelift. In fact, it is extremely rare. There is always some temporary loss of sensation in the skin of the face after surgery. This usually recovers within a few months.

Trauma to the greater auricular nerve may result in loss of sensation to the ear. This nerve is found below the ear, in the lateral part of the neck. Although injury to this nerve is very rare, if it is damaged it can lead to distressing sensations and pain around the ear, which may be difficult to treat.

More serious is the potential for damage to the facial nerve, which controls movement of facial muscles. Any competent facelift surgeon will have a thorough knowledge of the anatomy of this nerve and experience and training to avoid any injury or damage when carrying out the procedure. Occasionally, a branch of the nerve may be affected by swelling or bruising, but will quickly recover. Some very aggressive facelift techniques carry a higher risk of injury.

Delayed healing is also rare, and infection is very uncommon in the face. Minor delays in wound healing may be experienced but normally resolve within a few weeks.

A face lift *will*:

**!** clean and restore the jaw line

**!** remove loose skin and fat from the neck and under the chin

**!** soften the lines that run from the nose to the mouth.

A facelift *will not*:

**✗** improve the eye and forehead region

**✗** improve the lines and wrinkles around the lips and chin.

Ageing involves the whole face. To achieve a natural result, it is often necessary to carry out additional procedures to improve the eyes and brow area and the lines around the lips and chin. These include blepharoplasty, brow lift, fat transfer, and laser or chemical peels (see Chapter 10).

# Non-surgical 'facelifts'

## Peels, laser, and dermabrasion

There are several treatment modalities that may improve specific features of facial ageing without resorting to surgery. These are not very useful in reversing established gravitational changes, but can be effective in improving the smoothness and texture of facial skin.

At the most basic level, the health and appearance of skin will respond to improving diet, hydrating the skin by drinking plenty of water, avoiding excess sun, and stopping smoking. Modern anti-ageing skin creams contain active agents to moisturize and hydrate the skin and protect against sun damage. Antioxidants and exfoliants have also been shown to reduce the impact of skin toxins and to encourage the shedding of dead cells from the skin surface. It is likely that evolving technology will further advance the effectiveness of anti-ageing creams. At the present time, there are a confusing plethora of skin creams with impressive claims and promises but little scientific evidence to substantiate them.

In youth, the dead cells that form the outer layer of the skin are shed and replaced by new cells. Ageing skin is slower to repair itself. It also becomes thinner and may develop pigment changes (sun spots) and broken capillaries (fine red veins).

Improvement in texture and appearance of the skin can be achieved with the use of 'peeling' agents. Essentially, these remove the outer layer of epidermal cells and stimulate cell turnover. Peeling the skin is possible with a variety of agents, varying in strength. Gentle peels are achieved with the use of a variety of mildly acidic agents. These include the so-called 'fruit' acid peels (citric and glycolic acids), collectively known as alpha-hydroxy acids. They may make the skin feel tighter and smoother and often improve very fine surface wrinkles. The effect is mild and temporary. More effective agents include a prescription medication containing retinoids.

Deeper stronger peels can be very effective in improving and softening wrinkles and removing brown 'sun spots'. They remove not only the outer 'epidermal' skin but also the top layer of the deeper skin structure known as the 'dermis'. Deeper peels result in more tissue damage and a longer recovery period. The skin may be red and 'raw' for up to 10 days. Careful attention to the peeled area is necessary to prevent infection, and scratching or picking the wound must be resisted. This type of peel is usually performed using varying strengths of trichloroacetic acid. The potential complications of this type of peeling include 'hypopigmentation' (permanent lighter or paler skin colour) and scarring.

The deepest peels are performed with phenol and croton oil. The effects can be dramatic but so is the injury to the skin. It often requires an anaesthetic as the skin reaction to the acid is very painful. Recovery takes up to 10 days and the skin may be red for several weeks. Peeled skin may also lose the ability to tan and further sun exposure is unwise.

Phenol peels are now used relatively rarely and should only be performed by experienced surgeons or dermatologists.

The basic principle of improving skin texture and tone by removing the outer skin layer can be achieved in other ways. Dermabrasion is a technique popular with many surgeons whereby the outer layer of the skin is mechanically removed using a high speed drill with a rotary 'brush'. Results and recovery are similar to that of medium peels. Peels or dermabrasion are not suitable for those:

- with a history of cold sores or 'herpes'

- with a tendency to form bad scars

- not prepared to avoid further sun exposure.

## Laser therapy

There is a general perception that laser treatment is little short of miraculous with an ability to easily correct a wide range of conditions. Their value and application is still evolving as advances in laser technology are still being developed. In many respects, lasers have the same effect as peels and dermabrasion, by removing outer layers of the skin. The difference is in the way the injury to the skin is achieved.

> LASER is an acronym for Light Amplification of Stimulated Emission of Radiation.

Essentially, light energy is converted into a beam of monochromatic radiation along various parts of the spectrum of wavelengths. This energy or heat can be delivered in a controlled manner at different wavelengths for specific purposes. So, energy targeted at the surface of the skin will coagulate and 'ablate' these tissues. Energy can also be directed to be absorbed by red or black tissues and vaporize tattoo pigment or broken veins. Some lasers are designed to deliver energy to deeper layers of the skin to destroy hair follicles. 'Ablative' laser therapy removes the surface skin cells elegantly and with a precise controlled amount of energy. In terms of improvement in skin quality and texture, the principle and method is similar to that of peels and dermabrasion.

Recent advances in laser technology have developed systems for delivery of energy to the deeper layers of the skin without damaging the surface layers. This has great appeal as it avoids the problems of a skin wound and the recovery period for the skin to heal itself.

The use of these non-ablative lasers in facial rejuvenation is based on the principle that the energy delivered to the deeper layers of the skin causes contraction and tightening of the skin structures and stimulates the growth of new fibroblasts and collagen. This should result in firmer and smoother skin. It has also been suggested that this treatment may treat jowls and loose neck skin, although these claims have not been clearly substantiated.

Other technologies claiming to tighten the deeper facial tissues and restore a youthful appearance include the use of radio-frequency waves (Thermage®) to deliver energy to the subcutaneous tissues of the face. The energy is claimed to tighten and lift the facial tissues. Although some patients do report benefit, a recent review of patients in the USA states that 70% of patients had little or no result from the treatment!

At the present time, most aesthetic surgeons are sceptical about the claims and efficacy of laser and radio-frequency therapies for established anatomical and gravitational features of ageing.

 **Patient's perspective**

Jane is 48 years old. She is a successful lawyer with two daughters aged 10 and 12. Her work colleagues are mostly in their thirties. She goes to the gym two or three times a week and feels fit and healthy. For a year or two, she has noticed her jaw line is not as smooth as it was and she has some loose skin in her neck. Friends and colleagues have started to tell her she looks 'tired'. She feels she looks older than other mothers at the school gates and is anxious that she is 'losing her looks'. When someone asks if she is her 10-year-old's grandmother, she decides to investigate the option of cosmetic surgery.

Using the internet, she discovers that there are an extensive number of sites providing cosmetic surgery. She wants to ensure that she will see an experienced and qualified surgeon who practises in a reputable hospital with modern facilities. After exploring the options, she identifies three surgeons who fulfil her criteria. They are fully trained plastic surgeons with a specific interest in facial cosmetic surgery. Their websites list their training, hospital appointments, and research and teaching profile.

She makes an appointment for a consultation with two surgeons in her area. At both consultations she is seen by the surgeon who will carry out the procedure. They both explore her medical history and her motivation for and expectations of surgery. After examining her face, they explain carefully the options, including the risks and complications. They also show her photographs of their results. They both provide written information and offer a second consultation should she wish to proceed.

She discusses the option of surgery with her husband and close friends. She returns for a second consultation with one of the surgeons. She has a list of pre-prepared questions regarding the procedure, aftercare, and follow-up. She specifically requests that she does not want to look 'stretched' and 'tight'. She seeks reassurance that the result will be natural.

Following this consultation, she feels confident and motivated to proceed with surgery. However, there are practical problems with deciding on a suitable time. 'Downtime' means time off work and avoiding social commitments. After some hesitation, she decides to tell her children she will be having 'some treatment' to her face that may make her look a little bruised and swollen for a week or two.

On the day of surgery she arrives at the hospital early in the morning, having had nothing to eat or drink since midnight. She is admitted by one of the nurses and is seen by the surgeon and the anaesthetist.

When she wakes up after the operation, she is back in her room. She is pleasantly surprised that there is no pain and she sleeps well. The following morning, she is seen again by her surgeon. The bandages and dressings are all removed. The surgeon is pleased with her progress and the nurses wash her hair. She is given instructions for the next few days and appointment times for her follow-up. She also has contact numbers if there are any problems and is given painkillers and antibiotics to take home.

Back home, she examines her face in the mirror. Although she is swollen with a little bruising around her neck, she is delighted to see her jaw line is smooth and she has no loose skin in her neck. For the next several days she has a restful time at home. She sleeps on three pillows and is careful to take all her medication. On the fifth day she returns to the surgeon's office and has some fine stitches removed from the incisions in front of her ears. The stitches behind her ears are removed at a second visit, 10 days after surgery. By this time, she can cover most of the bruising with makeup and feels confident enough to go shopping.

Two and a half weeks after surgery, most of the swelling and bruising has disappeared. Her scars are still a little red but concealed by her hairstyle. Her face still feels a little numb.

Her daughters were initially a little alarmed by her appearance but are now complimentary about her appearance.

Six weeks after her surgery, she attends a social function with many of her work colleagues. She feels confident and is delighted that several people comment on how well and fresh she looks. Some people ask if she has lost weight or changed her hairstyle. No one asks if she has had surgery.

Six months later, Jane's scars have faded and she is confident to wear her hair up. She is delighted with the results of her surgery.

# ❓ FAQ

**Q1** What is a facelift?

**A** A facelift is a surgical operation designed to reverse the effects of gravity that produce features of ageing. These include lax neck skin and accumulation of fat under the chin, 'jowls' that obscure a clean jaw line and make the face look longer, squarer and heavier, and heavy, deep lines running from the side of the nose to the side of the mouth. The high cheekbones of youth may also sag and lose volume.

**Q2** Will a facelift remove the wrinkles around my eyes and mouth area?

**A** No. A facelift can reverse the effects of gravity but has no real effect on skin texture and damage caused by excess sun exposure, smoking, and other environmental toxins.

**Q3** What can I do for these problems?

**A** The approach to facial rejuvenation should be holistic. Wrinkles and lines in the forehead and eyelid area may need treatment with Botox. Specific treatment for damaged, thinned, and wrinkled skin may include laser, chemical peels, dermabrasion, and topical creams, such as retinoids. General skin health to minimize the effect of sun exposure requires attention to diet and the use of effective anti-ageing creams, including sun protection factors and antioxidants.

**Q4** How long will a facelift last?

**A** Imagine you had an identical twin. If you have a facelift, you will always look better than your twin who has not had surgery. However, although the clock has been turned back, the ageing process continues. How fast this occurs depends on many factors, including genetics, diet, exercise, and skin care. The majority of patients undergoing a facelift in their fifties rarely opt for another one. For those who do wish to repeat the procedure, it is rarely requested less than 8–10 years after the first facelift.

Q5  At what age should or could I have a facelift?

A  These days, the largest group of women have surgery in their mid to late forties, although it can be performed for anyone between their late thirties to their seventies or even eighties.

Q6  What sort of facelift should I have?

A  There are many different types of facelift. Your surgeon should recommend a procedure based on a number of criteria, including your facial anatomy, skin type, facial volume, and general health. The relative benefits and limitations of any recommended operation should be carefully explained in relation to your own desires and expectations.

Q7  What kind of scars will I have?

A  Most facelifts will involve scars in front of and behind the ears. They are planned very carefully and are usually very discreet. It is often said that 'you can hide them from a lover but not from your hairdresser'. In some circumstances, the scar behind the ear can be avoided, the so-called 'short scar' techniques. Rarely, the 'volumetric' facelift' may avoid ear scars, being performed via cuts in the mouth and in the temporal hair line. These reduced scar techniques, however, are only suitable for a relatively small group of patients with specific facial ageing patterns.

Q8  How long will it take for me to return to work and resume my social life?

A  For almost all facelifts, an obligatory 'downtime' of 2–3 weeks is required. After 6 weeks, full social, professional, and sporting activity can be confidently resumed. For many months after this, the scars will continue to fade. During this time, you may not feel confident to wear your hair up.

Q9  What are the possible complications of the operation?

A  Bleeding, infection, and nerve damage are all possible. Infection is extremely rare as the blood supply to the face is excellent. Occasionally, some minor delay in healing may occur but this is usually temporary and rarely affects the recovery or the result. Nerve damage always causes some numbness in the cheeks, although this recovers within a month or two. More serious is the potential to damage the nerves responsible for facial movement, including raising the eyebrows and moving the lips. Fortunately, in the hands of an experienced facial surgeon, this is extremely rare. If weakness of facial muscles does occur, it is generally as a result of bruising to the nerve, which recovers within a time frame of a few days to a month or so. Bleeding into the face after surgery is a recognized complication and may affect 2–3% of all cases. Risk factors for bleeding have been identified and include:

♦ smoking

♦ pre-existing untreated high blood pressure

♦ ingestion of aspirin and anti-inflammatory painkillers such as ibuprofen.

Bleeding is also more common in men. The key to managing a postoperative bleed is rapid diagnosis and treatment. Bleeding causes pain and swelling in the side of the face. Once recognized by nursing staff, the surgical team are informed and recalled. Once the diagnosis is confirmed, the treatment involves rapid return to the operating theatre where the blood clot is removed. Following prompt treatment, recovery is then usually uneventful.

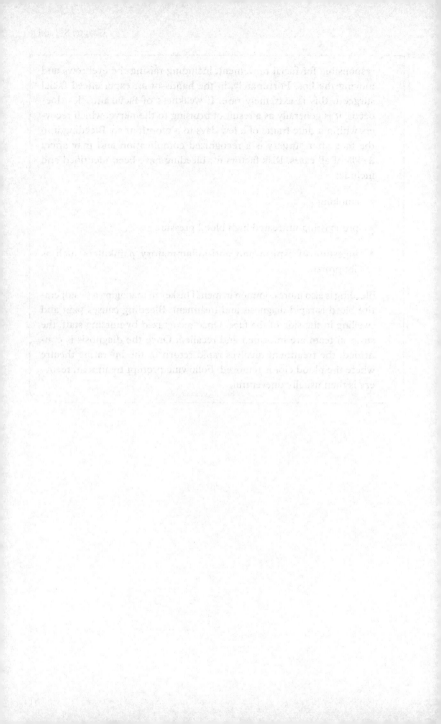

# 9

# Rhinoplasty

## ➲ Key points

◆ The nose must be assessed with regard to the whole face including the brow and the chin.

◆ Surgery to improve the appearance of the nose must preserve the function of the nose.

◆ Modern rhinoplasty tends to modify existing structures rather than remove them.

◆ Surgeon and patient must agree on realistic expectations of what can or cannot be achieved.

Rhinoplasty (a nose job) is a popular procedure. The nose is a prominent and highly visible feature of the face and has a powerful impact on our perception of attractiveness. If the nose appears to be to long, prominent, thick, thin, bulbous, wide, pointy, crooked, or droopy, surgery may be considered. The problem may be confined to one area such as the tip of the nose or a pronounced 'hump'. If the problem is due to a bent or crooked nose, this may be due to previous trauma or injury. Often this may result in a variety of 'functional' problems, including breathing difficulty, snoring, excessive mucus, blockages, and allergic-type symptoms. The surgery for these problems may involve a 'septoplasty' and/or a 'turbinectomy', which may or may not normally be required as part of an operation to improve appearance.

In the right circumstances, a rhinoplasty can dramatically improve the aesthetics of the nose and the whole face. The goal of the operation should be to produce an attractive nose that suits the face, providing harmony and balance. It is often said that the nose should be 'silent' on the face and allow other facial characteristics (for example, the eyes) to be appreciated. It is very important to understand the limitations of rhinoplasty and to appreciate what can and cannot be done. It is also essential to appreciate that surgery will not automatically result in social, sexual, and professional success!

It follows that in the assessment of anyone considering a rhinoplasty, careful analysis of the whole face is essential. This must include the prominence or strength of the chin, the width and height of the face, and the distance between the eyes.

There are some generally accepted measurements that act as a guide for the ideal relationship between the nose and the rest of the face. These are often condensed in the so-called 'rule of thirds' (Figure 9.1).

There are differences in the generally accepted ideals for the shape of the male and female nose. A female nose should have a straight dorsum with a tip that gently projects from the dorsum. A male nose is generally straighter throughout the whole length of the nose. Each individual will have their own

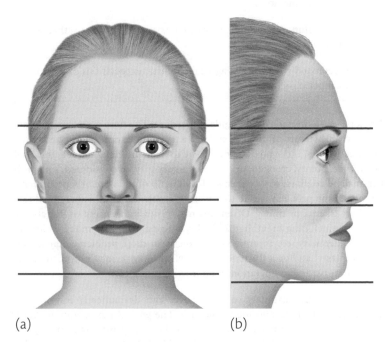

(a)                                    (b)

**Figure 9.1** Face (a) frontal and (b) in profile to show the rule of thirds.

facial dimensions and characteristics that determine the scope and outcome of a rhinoplasty.

Ethnic origin may also influence the nature of surgery and there are specific procedures designed for Asian and Afro-Caribbean noses, to augment the dorsal profile or reduce naturally wide nostrils. Thick scarring may occur a little more often in certain ethnic groups and should be taken into consideration.

For any patient, there are some circumstances that limit the potential for a positive outcome. These include:

- thick sebaceous nasal skin—this may always mask the features of the underlying structures and their definition, however exquisite

- a history of poor scarring

- unrealistic expectations

- emotional or psychological instability.

## The consultation

As with any proposed surgical procedure, a full medical history should be reviewed to establish general health and psychological stability. Specific enquiry relating to the nose should include:

- allergies, sinusitis, previous injuries or fractures, breathing difficulties, snoring

- recreational drug use, specifically cocaine.

The surgeon should explore the motivation for surgery and the features of the nose that are perceived as undesirable. Critically, the expectations and goals of the procedure must be established.

Examination of the nose should include an assessment of the whole face noting any asymmetry, normal relationship of the upper and lower jaws, prominence of the chin, cheekbones, forehead, and height and volume of the upper lip. The surgeon should record:

- whether the skin of the nose is thick, oily, thin, or papery

- whether the nose is straight

- what part of the nose is bone and what part is cartilage

- whether the cartilage is stiff, springy, or soft and weak

- if there is air entry in both nostrils

- if the nostrils are wide or narrow

- the width, length, and projection of the nose

- the presence of a 'hump' and position of the tip—upturned, long and droopy, or retracted.

- the width and support of the middle of the nose.

Successful rhinoplasty can be achieved if:

- the patient can clearly identify the features of their nose they wish to change

- the surgeon broadly agrees with the patient's assessment

- the surgeon is confident that the desired changes can be achieved and will produce a more aesthetic nose that is appropriate for the face

- the patient accepts that there are limitations to surgery and perfection may not be possible.

Rhinoplasty is unlikely to be successful if:

- the patient perceives abnormal features of the nose that are vague or minimal

- the patient has a fixed idea of the nose they want, often chosen from an individual celebrity, which is unrealistic or inappropriate

- the patient believes that rhinoplasty will improve career prospects, and social and sexual success.

Occasionally, rhinoplasty may be sought by individuals with severe psychological or psychiatric disorders. In the USA, several surgeons have been injured or killed by prospective (predominantly male) patients.

Although not infallible, there is a maxim for surgeons to describe unsuitable patients for rhinoplasty—SIMON!

SIMON stands for Single, Immature, Male, and Overly Narcissistic.

# The operation

It is probably true to say that in the field of cosmetic surgery, the philosophy and nature of rhinoplasty has changed more than for any other procedure over the last 20 years. A better understanding of the anatomy and function of the nose has led to an appreciation that simply removing tissue is at best simplistic and at worst very damaging.

Bone and cartilage in the nose not only determines shape but also provides support for the nose to ensure free airflow during normal breathing and when demand is increased by exercise. Removing too much tissue can result in a short, scooped, or collapsed flat nose. The appearance may often worsen with time. Also, breathing difficulties can result from weakening the internal structure of the nose called the nasal 'valves'. Even if the function is not affected, the nose may have an 'operated' or 'done' look, which is no longer viewed as desirable.

Modern rhinoplasty still includes techniques to reduce or remove some tissue, but these are balanced by others, which seek to modify or reconfigure tissues with an emphasis on preserving essential features and function. Although it seems unlikely, many rhinoplasty procedures actually involve adding tissue in the form of grafts, to ensure support and a natural look to the nose.

The procedure can be performed with two different approaches, either 'closed' or 'open'. The closed approach is performed through an incision placed within the nose, which may limit the exposure or visibility of the nasal structures during the operation. An open approach involves the placement of an incision that runs across the columella at the base of the nose as a 'V' or a step (Figure 9.2). This allows the surgeon to lift the skin and soft tissues of the nose and provides an extremely good view of the underlying cartilages and other structures. There are different reasons for choosing between these approaches and excellent results can be achieved with both. Experienced surgeons will often carry out both types of approach depending on the needs of individual cases. Either way, the surgery is performed under general anaesthetic and may take between 1 and 3 hours.

The tip of the nose can be made smaller by removing cartilage in this area. A wide tip can be narrowed by changing the shape or position of these cartilages. If the tip is drooping, it can be shortened and lifted by using cartilage grafts to support the tip in its new position. Reducing the projection of the nose and removing a hump is usually achieved by removing cartilage from the septum and some of the nasal bone. When the profile is straight, the nose may need to be

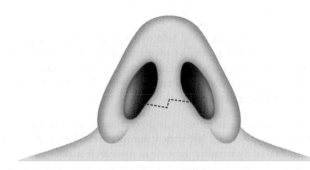

**Figure 9.2** Open rhinoplasty trans-columella incision.

narrowed to balance the other changes. This requires a controlled fracture (break) to narrow the nasal bones. Although this is often performed through an incision inside the nose, some surgeons prefer to use tiny incisions in the skin on the side of the nose. These heal very quickly and are virtually invisible after a few weeks.

To achieve a natural and attractive result, small pieces of cartilage may be added to the tip, sides, and dorsum of the nose. These grafts are usually taken from within the nose itself. Occasionally, extra cartilage may be needed and can be taken from the ear or even the ribs. This is rarely necessary for most rhinoplasties but is useful when the nose needs to be rebuilt or restored. If the tip area of the nose is too wide, the nostrils can be narrowed by removing small wedges of tissue at the base of the nose. The incisions are placed around the base of the nostril and the scars are usually not visible.

> The techniques used to produce an attractive, natural result have to be tailored to suit individual circumstances. Rhinoplasty surgeons must have the ability and experience to assess and analyse the problem and plan a bespoke procedure.

At the end of the operation, the nose is protected from unwanted movement and swelling with the use of a splint or plaster as well as surgical tape. Packing the nostrils with gauze is no longer routinely performed and the absence of packs has greatly reduced the degree of discomfort postoperatively.

Indeed, most patients experience little or no pain during the recovery period. To minimize swelling, it is often recommended that patients sleep in a semi-sitting position for several days.

## Postoperative care

The splint is removed 7–10 days after surgery. At this stage, the shape and size of the new nose can be appreciated. However, further refinement will occur as the internal swelling resolves. This process can take up to 3 months! During this time, it is quite normal for the nose to be a little congested. There may be some numbness of the skin, particularly in the tip area. The skin may also have a tendency to appear red and inflamed from time to time. This often occurs after alcohol, exercise, stress, and temperature change, and may persist for some months.

Flying should be avoided for 4 weeks as during this time the nose may become easily congested and nose bleeds can occur. Vigorous exercise and contact sports should be avoided for 6 weeks after surgery. At this time, any breaks in the bones of the nose will be healed and as strong as before surgery. Six months after surgery, the final result is achieved and all swelling will have disappeared.

It is generally accepted that 5% of all cases may require some form of secondary adjustment to correct any minor contour irregularities or asymmetries.

### ⓘ Patient's perspective

Anne is 28 years old. She has been married for 4 years and has a 2-year-old daughter. She works as an accounts manager for a large publishing company.

From the age of 14, she has hated the shape of her nose. Although it looks fine from the front, on profile she has a large 'hump' and the tip of the nose is 'droopy' and long. She thinks she looks like a witch! Anxiety about her nose has waxed and waned, but she has always avoided photographs and takes care to avoid presenting her profile whenever possible. She insisted on previewing her wedding photographs and discarded more than two-thirds of them because she thought her nose was too prominent.

She had considered the option of surgery for many years, but was dissuaded by her friends and family. They always said her nose was 'strong' and 'had character'.

A female work colleague returned from a 2-week holiday and revealed she had had a 'nose job'. Anne was amazed by the result and resolved to follow suit. She asked her friend for the surgeon's contact number and rang to make an appointment the same day.

Her husband was supportive of her decision and accompanied her to the consultation. They were both impressed by the surgeon and his thorough explanation of the procedure. He showed them examples of his results with photographs of other patients he had treated. Anne was relieved that the surgeon thought her request was reasonable and achievable.

She wanted to book a date for surgery there and then but the surgeon insisted she take some time to reflect on the information he provided. He suggested a second consultation (with no additional consultation fee) in a few weeks' time. Anne felt completely committed to surgery and her only anxiety was that the surgeon would change his mind. Before the second consultation, she spent a lot of time researching the operation and her surgeon on the internet. She was reassured to discover that her surgeon was often invited to lecture at meetings and teach on courses on the subject of rhinoplasty.

After the second consultation, Anne booked a date for surgery! Having made the decision, she wanted to have the operation as soon as possible.

A few days before her admission, she experienced some feelings of doubt. She wondered if she was being frivolous and self-indulgent—Should she use her money in this way? Her husband reminded her that this was something she had always wanted and encouraged her to proceed. She did.

Ten days after the operation, she went to the surgeon's office with a combination of excitement and anxiety. This was the day when the plaster would be removed and she would see her new nose for the first time. Anne would always remember the moment when she looked in the mirror. Although her nose felt swollen and a little numb, she was amazed at the result. The hump had gone. The new nose was everything she had hoped for. Her eyes seemed so big!

# ❓ FAQ

Q1 What are the risks of rhinoplasty?

A The operation itself is very safe and there are few risks to your general health. Dissatisfaction with the result is the biggest problem. Sometimes this can reflect poor communication with the surgeon as to the anticipated outcome. Even with a good result, there can be a transitional period where the new appearance is settling. Swelling can take some months to resolve before the final effect is appreciated. Occasionally, practical or functional problems can be produced if too much tissue is removed. These problems include breathing difficulties, or an 'overdone' look. Also, the skin of the nose may sometimes appear reddish due to broken blood vessels (telangiectasia).

Q2 My daughter is desperate to have a rhinoplasty but she is only 16. Should she wait until she is older?

A Until relatively recently, it was thought that operating on the nose in the teenage years might interfere with subsequent growth of the nose. It is now appreciated that this is not true and rhinoplasty can safely be performed from early teenage. However, at this age suitability and psychological maturity are the most important considerations.

Q3 I had always believed that rhinoplasty left no scars on the skin of the nose, but my surgeon says I will have a scar at the base of my nose and small scars on the sides. Is this really necessary?

A Rhinoplasty can be performed through incisions concealed entirely within the nose. This is known as an 'endonasal' rhinoplasty. However, in many circumstances, a surgeon may opt for a different approach using an incision across the columella at the base of the middle of the nostrils. This is called an 'open' rhinoplasty. Also, some surgeons break the nose using tiny incisions on the side of the nose where the nose meets the cheek. If the nostrils are very wide, further incisions may be placed around the base of the nostrils. All these scars generally heal very well and are barely visible after a few months.

Q4 I really want a rhinoplasty as my nose is quite thick and fleshy. I saw a surgeon who refuses to operate as he says that the main problem is that I have thick skin on my nose and surgery will not help. Surely something can be done?

A Any responsible and experienced surgeon will carefully assess all elements of the nose before deciding to operate. These include cartilage, bone, and skin. Unfortunately, there are few options for refining the nose if the skin is very thick. Thick skin does not re-drape well on the underlying cartilage and bone and the results of surgery are often disappointing.

Q5 I had a rhinoplasty 2 months ago and love the result. However, my nose is still stuffy, especially in the mornings and sometimes can be a little runny. Is this normal?

A It is not unusual for the nose to feel a little blocked or stuffy many months after surgery. This is often worse at certain times such as after exercise or in a smoky environment. The stuffiness should gradually improve and disappear but it may take up to a year.

Q6 I went to a surgeon to get my nose done and he said I should have an operation to enhance (augment) my chin at the same time. Is this a good idea?

A The idea of a rhinoplasty is to produce an attractive nose that is in balance with the rest of the face. If the chin is retrusive or weak, a rhinoplasty alone may not achieve this balance. Genioplasty is frequently offered to patients seeking rhinoplasty for this reason.

Q7 I had a rhinoplasty 15 years ago when I was 22 years old. I liked the result at the time. Over the years, however, I now think it looks very obvious that I have had a nose job. The nose is very pinched and I have a lot of difficulty breathing, particularly at night. When I breathe in sharply, the tip of my nose collapses inwards and I can't breathe at all! Can I rectify this problem?

A Fashion changes and so does surgical technique. In the past, surgeons often carried out rhinoplasties that relied on removing tissue for the effect. Regrettably, it is now accepted that this may result in a loss of support for the nose that has a 'stigmatic' appearance and that functional problems may result. Secondary or revisional rhinoplasty is an option and can be very successful but requires a high level of surgical skill and experience. The procedure frequently involves putting cartilage back into the nose to rebuild and strengthen the tissues.

# 10

# Eyelid and brow surgery

## ➲ Key points

◆ Eyelid surgery is complex and demanding. The surgeon should be highly skilled and experienced in these techniques.

◆ Lower eyelid surgery has the potential to cause a variety of problems that are difficult to correct.

◆ The eyelid area must be treated in the context of the rest of the face.

Ageing in the upper third of the face affects the brow, upper and lower eyelids, and the cheek area. These structures are not improved by a traditional facelift, which is directed at the lower cheek, jowls, jaw line, and neck. This distinction is very important to understand for several reasons. As well as appreciating the scope of facelifting by itself, it also explains why the results of facelifting may be disappointing. A facelift may achieve its objectives but result in a imbalance or disharmony in the overall effect. The features of ageing in the upper face may even be accentuated.

The features of a youthful eye are well understood (see Figure 10.1). For the lower lid:

◆ the lid is convex (bows outwards)

◆ the lashes are full and everted (turned outward)

◆ the lid should rise higher at the lateral corner than at the medial corner

◆ the skin should be smooth with no wrinkles

◆ the lid should describe a gentle 'S' curve

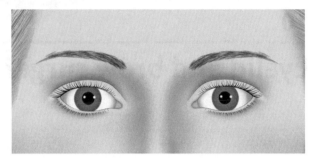

**Figure 10.1** Youthful eye area.

♦ there should be a smooth transition between the lid and the cheek

♦ the lid should cover the lower 1–2 mm of the pupil.

With age, the skin may become lax and wrinkles appear, often worse in smokers and with cumulative sun damage. Hyperpigmentation (dark circles), spidery blood vessels, and brown 'sunspots' may also develop. Pockets of fat may become more prominent and produce 'bags' under the lower eyelid. The cheek tissues often drop, which makes the lower eyelid look longer and accentuates a deep circle or 'tear trough'. Increased laxity or looseness of the lid itself may result in the lid drooping, which conveys a look of tiredness and sadness. In the upper lid, ageing may result in:

♦ the lid being hidden by folds of excess skin

♦ descent of the eyebrow.

These changes tend to hide the eyes and make them appear smaller. It is increasingly difficult to apply makeup. In extreme cases, the folds of extra skin may even interfere with vision.

Given the importance of the eyes to our overall appearance, it is not surprising that cosmetic eyelid surgery is a frequently requested and popular procedure. It is estimated that 50 000 blepharoplasty procedures are performed every year in the USA.

There is a generally held view that eyelid surgery is simple, quick and effective. However, as with all procedures, expert assessment and analysis of the anatomical changes is essential and the surgery must be tailored to suit each individual. Features of ageing in the upper third of the face (see Figure 10.2) include:

* brow descent (the eyebrow drops)

* dermatochalasis (extra skin folds)

* reduction of upper lid show (the extra skin rests on the lashes)

* lateral hooding (the extra skin may cover the outer part of the eye).

Features of ageing in the lower eyelid include:

* tear trough (a groove under the eyelid where it joins the cheek)

* prominent fat bags

* malar bags (fluid-filled pouches under the eyelid)

* lateral canthal descent (the outer part of the eye drops downwards)

* skin changes (see below)

* lengthening of the lid–cheek junction (the eyelid area looks longer as the cheek tissue drops)

* skeletal reveal (loss of fat in the face shows the bones around the eye area)

* lid laxity (the eyelid becomes loose and floppy).

Skin changes include the appearances of:

* lines

* dyschromias (brown spots)

* actinic damage

* telangiectasias (spidery red blood vessels).

Until relatively recently, cosmetic surgery to the eyelids, known as blepharoplasty, involved the removal of skin, fat, and muscle. This approach usually improved the appearance of ageing eyelids, but for many patients could result in significant functional problems and a stigmatic or operated look. It is now appreciated that simply removing tissue is not always appropriate.

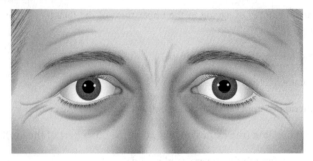

**Figure 10.2** Aged eye area.

Advances in the understanding of eyelid anatomy have led to the development of new approaches, designed to preserve a natural appearance and avoid complications. Standard blepharoplasty has the potential to cause a number of problems including:

* scleral show—the white of the eye can be seen under the pupil as the lid descends

* lid malposition—the lids may rest in different positions after surgery

* rounding of the eye

* hollowing

* descent of the lateral canthus—the outer part of the eye drops downwards giving a sad droopy look to the eye

* an operated look

* loss of vision or blindness after blepharoplasty—an extremely remote but appalling possibility.

After any blepharoplasty, it may be normal to experience swelling, bruising, excess watering, grittiness, or itching. Occasionally, the eyelid may drop, exposing the white of the eye underneath the pupil (the 'sclera') to produce scleral show.

To achieve a more natural result, modern techniques include:

* preserving fat and skin

* supporting the lid

* repositioning rather than removing tissue.

Crucially, it is now appreciated that correction of the features of the ageing lower eyelid must include the changes that affect the cheek or midface area.

Careful assessment and analysis of any patient requesting eyelid surgery should include:

- a history of dry or gritty eyes

- excessive watering of the eye

- a history of thyroid problems

- intolerance of contact lens use

- collagen or autoimmune disorders

- kidney disease

- bleeding disorders

- redness or burning of the eyelids

- psychiatric disorders

- alcohol, tobacco, and steroid use

- previous eye surgery

- family history of glaucoma

- visual impairment.

The presence of one or more of these may influence the decision to proceed with surgery.

## Upper lid blepharoplasty

The development of folds of skin in the upper eyelid contribute to a tired and aged look. It can be difficult or impossible to apply makeup. The excess skin may rest on the eyelashes or even hang over the eye and impair vision. With increasing age, the skin may become loose and 'baggy'. The appearance of excess skin may also be a result of drooping and descent of the eyebrow and forehead.

Surgery can be extremely effective in correcting these problems and restoring a natural youthful appearance. If the eyebrow is in a normal position, an upper blepharoplasty is normally performed. If the brow has descended, a more natural result may involve a brow lift. Occasionally, both procedures may be indicated.

Upper blepharoplasty involves the removal of excess skin and muscle from the upper lid. After removal of the excess tissue, the wound is closed with fine stitches. The stitch line and subsequent scar are placed in a natural fold or skin crease (Figure 10.3).

If the eyebrow has dropped, a better result may be achieved by performing a 'brow lift'. This is usually performed with 'keyhole' or endoscopic surgery, using a camera and specially designed instruments. The incisions are small and placed behind the hairline in the scalp.

Upper blepharoplasty can be performed with a local anaesthetic and can be an outpatient procedure, whereas a brow lift usually requires a general anaesthetic and an overnight stay in hospital.

# Brow lift

To achieve a natural appearance in the brow and eyelid area (the upper third of the face or 'periorbital' area) it may be necessary to lift the eyebrow area. The eyebrow descends with age and the skin of the brow becomes looser and lined. This can result in hooding of the skin in the outer lid area and the eye itself appears smaller or hidden.

The surgical procedures for lifting the brow have become more sophisticated and less invasive. Originally, an incision was required across the scalp from ear to ear (the open or 'coronal' approach). This has been superseded by the

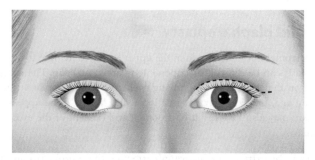

**Figure 10.3** Upper eye incisions.

advent of endoscopic (keyhole) techniques. Using surgical telescopes and cameras, brow lift can be performed through three or four small incisions hidden in the scalp. The brow tissue is lifted and fixed in position to the bone of the forehead (Figure 10.4).

Recovery is much quicker although mild swelling and bruising is usual. The operation may also produce some numbness in the scalp for several weeks. Hair loss in and around the incision area is frequently cited as a complication of brow surgery. However, this is very rare (less than 1%), and may be the result of medication or an individual response to stress. Hair is not shaved or cut for the operation. Some dryness or thinning of the hair has been reported but this is temporary.

Another potential complication is asymmetry. It is important to determine whether the eyebrows are symmetrical before surgery as this is quite common.

The open brow lift often resulted in a higher hairline, a problem avoided with the endoscopic brow lift. However, in the first week or two after the operation, it is normal for the brow to look a little high and feel tight and stiff.

Brow lift can be extremely successful in restoring a natural, fresh appearance. It is important that the surgeon avoids lifting the eyebrow too much, which

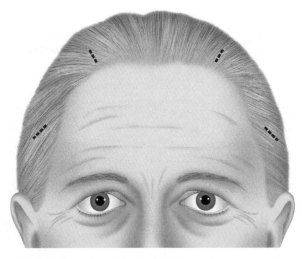

**Figure 10.4** Incisions for endocscopic brow lift.

may cause a 'surprised' look The aim of a brow lift is to produce an attractive shape to the brow, often with a graceful arch towards the outer third of the eyebrow. A modification of brow lift surgery is a procedure that concentrates on this area, the so-called 'lateral brow lift' or temporal lift.

# Lower lid blepharoplasty

Surgery to rejuvenate the ageing lower eyelid is more complicated than for the upper lid and the recovery time is longer. There are several different operations including:

◆ *Transconjuctival blepharoplasty.* This procedure removes or repositions prominent fat bags through a cut on the inside of the eyelid. It is popular as it leaves no scar on the skin and recovery is usually quite quick.

◆ *Subciliary approach.* A more traditional approach requiring a cut along the margin of the eyelid (Figure 10.5). This is required when removal of excess skin from the lid is required. A 'canthopexy' is often included. This involves a stitch in the corner of the lid to lift the margin of the lid or to ensure that the lid does not drop or retract after surgery.

◆ A more complex operation may aim to *reposition excess fat rather than remove it and lift and re-drape the muscles of the eyelid and cheek area.* This can be very successful if performed by a surgeon with special training and experience.

◆ Excess skin in the lower lid can be tightened and improved using *laser or chemical peels.* However, these techniques may cause hypopigmentation of

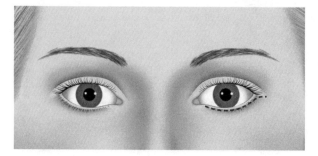

**Figure 10.5** The subciliary incision for lower blepahroplasty.

the skin with a permanent pale colour. Conversely, the skin may darken and appear brown as hyperpigmentation may also occur.

◆ *Midface lift.* If the appearance of an ageing lower eyelid is a result of sagging cheek tissues, improvement may require lifting of the cheek or midface. This can be achieved by several methods but all involve more radical and extensive surgery and often a long recovery period.

◆ *Fat grafting or fillers.* Early signs of ageing in the lower lid are usually identified by the appearance of a hollow or dark ring under the eyelid. The lid can be smoothed out in this area by injecting fat or a synthetic filler into the groove or hollow. This procedure requires care to avoid irregularities and lumpiness.

## Conclusions

It should be appreciated that cosmetic surgery on or around the eyelids is not simple and straightforward. Although it is popular and can be very effective, a successful, natural result requires a detailed, thorough and expert assessment of the problem and may a carefully chosen and executed procedure. A poor result can be difficult to correct and may cause distress, regret, recrimination, and litigation. Successful surgery requires a surgeon with training and experience and a patient with realistic expectations. There is no perfect eyelid operation and no perfect eyelid surgeon!

---

## ❷ Patient's perspective

Ellen is 43 years old and works for an advertising agency where most of the other people in her office are in their twenties. She has always been happy with her appearance and was at first surprised and then upset when several people asked her if she had had a late night or was feeling tired.

After a social function, photographs of the event were posted on the office notice board. This was the first time that Ellen realized that she really did look tired and that the problem was her eyelids! The bathroom mirror confirmed that she had developed folds of skin in the upper eyelid area, which had covered up the normal crease in the eyelid. This was why applying makeup had become more difficult in the last year or two. Ellen had bought some expensive eye cream (over £180 for a small pot!), and also read that drinking lots of water, avoiding alcohol, sleeping well, and avoiding stress would help. Her job and lifestyle were going to make this difficult.

After a few months, nothing had really changed. Ellen decided to consider cosmetic surgery. One of her oldest friends was a doctor, and Ellen called her for advice. Although her friend was a paediatrician, she offered to enquire within the medical community to find a recommended plastic surgeon. After a few days, she called back with the names of two surgeons. One was a plastic surgeon and the other was an eye surgeon (ophthalmologist)—both specialized in the eye and brow area and had an excellent reputation for cosmetic eyelid surgery.

Ellen's friend also told her that the operation was usually done under a local anaesthetic and could be done as an outpatient day case.

As it turned out, Ellen was surprised and a little upset by the advice and recommendations of both the surgeons! At both her consultations, she was told that although she would benefit from an upper blepharoplasty, the position of her eyebrow was low and the lateral eye area would still appear 'hooded' if only a blepharoplasty was performed.

Ellen was disappointed at first as she was hoping for a minimal procedure with a very quick recovery. However, a simple demonstration convinced her that the brow lift option was preferable. By placing two fingers above the eyebrow and gently lifting the skin, her whole eyelid and brow area looked so much better and fresher. The shape of her eyebrow also seemed much more feminine.

The upper eyelid blepharoplasty and endoscopic brow lift would require a general anaesthetic and an overnight stay in hospital. Downtime before returning to work would involve a week off work. Ellen waited until the approach of the Christmas holidays to book her surgery.

The practice nurse explained what to expect in the immediate postoperative period. When she came round from the anaesthetic, her eyes were covered with eyepad dressings. She could imagine that unprepared, it could be a little frightening to wake up and not be able to see! The eyepads were taken off a few hours after surgery although a coolpack was applied intermittently overnight. This helped to reduce swelling and bruising around the eyes.

The next morning, her hair was washed before leaving the hospital. Ellen was pleased that the swelling and bruising seemed to be very mild although her eyebrows seemed very tight and stiff. Also, her scalp felt rather numb. Within the scalp were four small incisions closed with metal clips. The scar in her eyelids was very fine and hidden in the crease.

For several days, she slept with her head elevated on three pillows. The eyelid stitches were removed after 3 days and the clips at 10 days. By then, her eyebrows had regained normal movement and the eyelid scars were barely visible. She was now free to use makeup.

When she returned to work, none of her colleagues knew she had had surgery but several commented on how well she looked and how fresh she looked after a holiday! The numbness was the only reminder of the surgery and this gradually disappeared after a few months.

## ❓ FAQ

Q1 I have an overactive thyroid and my eyelids have become puffy and fatty. Am I a candidate for blepharoplasty?

A Thyroid disease can produce very specific problems in and around the eye area that involves the eye muscles as well as the fat and skin. It is essential that the underlying thyroid condition is properly treated. Also, before any surgery is contemplated a thorough investigation and assessment of the eyes must be performed by an ophthalmologist. Surgery can be helpful but it requires a level of expertise for this specific condition.

Q2 My eyelids have lots of wrinkles, which look worse when I smile. Will surgery get rid of them?

A No. Wrinkles are produced by sun damage (static wrinkles) and the effect of contraction of the underlying muscles (dynamic wrinkles). Preventing further damage is possible using a skin cream with a strong sun protection factor. Botox is probably the best option for reducing the wrinkles, particularly if they are of the 'dynamic' type.

Q3  I have been told I need a 'canthopexy' as part of my lower eyelid blepharoplasty. What is this and why do I need it?

 A  One of the problems of lower blepharoplasty is that the eyelid can drop into a lower position after surgery. This can result from the pull of a scar on the delicate tissues of the lid. It can also happen if too much skin is removed. If the lid does drop, the eye can develop a rather round appearance, which gives a tired or sad look. It can also result in excessive or inappropriate watering or soreness. In order to prevent this from happening, many surgeons use a canthopexy at the same time as the blepharoplasty. This is essentially a supporting stitch placed at the corner of the eye. It can produce a rather slanted, almond shape to the eye in the first few weeks after surgery but this soon settles.

Q4  I have swellings of fluid underneath my eye area at the top of my cheek. Will surgery remove these?

 A  These swellings are known as malar oedema. Their cause is unknown but there is often a genetic predisposition. Surgery does not reliably remove them and, indeed, may make them worse! There is some evidence that an operation on the eyelid that releases and re-drapes the muscles around the eye can help. However, this procedure may require a long recovery period and is not foolproof. The degree of swelling can be minimized by avoiding nicotine, caffeine, and alcohol.

Q5  I have noticed that one of my eyes is droopier than the other one. Can surgery make them both equal?

 A  Some degree of difference between the eyes and the eyelid skin is almost inevitable and surgery can often help to make the appearance more symmetrical. However, it is possible that you may have another condition affecting the droopy eye, called 'ptosis'. Careful examination by your surgeon should diagnose this condition. It is very important that the presence of ptosis is recognized as traditional cosmetic surgery will not be effective. The problem with a droopy or 'ptotic' eyelid is caused by a problem with a muscle in the upper eyelid that is responsible for opening the eyelid. Ptosis can be corrected but requires a completely different surgical technique. You may need to be referred to an ophthalmic surgeon with special experience in this condition.

# 11

# Genioplasty

➡ **Key points**

◆ Surgeons offering genioplasty should have expertise in the normal and abnormal features of the facial bones, including the jaws.

◆ Suitability for chin augmentation must be determined by an expert analysis of the bones and soft tissues of the whole face.

◆ Genioplasty is often performed with a rhinoplasty to improve facial balance.

◆ Chin implants, although popular and simple, may produce a range of short- and long-term complications.

◆ Numbness of the lower lip is a possible complication of genioplasty.

◆ 'Simple' procedures such as the use of injectable fillers may only be temporary.

◆ Genioplasty, properly performed, provides a predictable, stable, and natural result.

The shape and size of the chin has an important impact on facial appearance. The forehead, nose, and chin should be balanced and harmonious. A small, retruded, or 'weak' chin may make the nose appear prominent or the lower lip pendulous, whereas a strong chin is seen as an important element of an attractive male face.

Augmenting the chin is a relatively popular procedure and can be achieved by a wide range of techniques, ranging from the use of injectable fillers to meticulously planned complex operations to move the mandible (lower jaw). The key to successful results is that the treatment should be determined by an expert assessment of the whole face and the relationship between the major segments of the facial bones. There are several established formulas or 'rules' that can be used to identify the causes of facial imbalance or abnormality. These include the relationship between the upper and lower jaws and the 'occlusion' or 'bite' patterns of the teeth. They also assess the position and measurements of the forehead, cheekbones, nose, lips, and chin. This assessment process is essential, as failure to accurately diagnose the facial elements responsible for an abnormality may lead to inappropriate treatment and a poor result. Therefore, any cosmetic surgeon undertaking this type of problem should be experienced in facial analysis and work closely with orthodontic or maxillofacial colleagues. The normal jaw is shown in Figure 11.1.

When it has been established that the primary problem is a small or retruded chin, a range of procedures can be considered. These include:

◆ *Plumping the soft tissue of the chin with injectable 'fillers'*. A range of materials have been used for this purpose including collagen, hyaluronic acid (Restylane and Perlane), hydroxyapatite pastes, silicone, and collagen fillers like Artecoll.

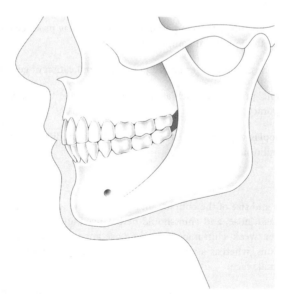

**Figure 11.1** Normal jaw.

- *Fat grafting.* This option is increasing in popularity. The fat is taken from the abdomen or thigh. It is then prepared by removing excess fluid and oils and injected into the chin.

- *Inserting a chin implant.* These may be manufactured in a range of sizes or as a 'block' that can be sculpted. Common materials include solid silicone and polyethylene. Some implants are designed for the chin area but others may be more extensive and can be used to increase the jaw line as well.

- *Bone grafting.* This technique involves harvesting bone from another part of the body (including the hip and skull) and grafting it on to the bone of the chin. It is usually secured in place by metal screws.

- *Chin advancement (genioplasty).* Experienced facial surgeons usually prefer this option. It involves cutting the bone of the chin and moving it forwards. It is secured in position with small screws or metal plates (Figures 11.2 and 11.3).

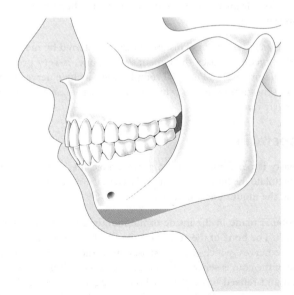

**Figure 11.2** Bone segment moved in genioplasty.

# Complications

For suitable candidates, a genioplasty can deliver an excellent result, with a dramatic improvement in facial balance and aesthetics. It is said that the improvement is virtually immediate and permanent. However, as with all surgery, there are potential complications. These are specific to the method employed. They can be summarized as follows:

- *Fillers.* Many are temporary and will be resorbed after 4–6 months. The permanent fillers have a greater risk of long-term problems including lumpiness, irregularity, and inflammatory reactions.

- *Fat grafting* has the advantage of using the patient's own tissue. Infection is rare although, as with fillers, the fat may be resorbed and the degree of resorption is unpredictable.

- *Chin implants* are popular as the surgery is relatively simple and the recovery period is short. However, they may produce a range of problems including infection, migration, and extrusion, and they may also cause erosion of the existing bone of the chin.

- *Bone grafting* is now infrequently used. It involves the extra surgery of taking bone from elsewhere and, over time, the bone may resorb or even disappear.

- *Advancement genioplasty.* This procedure is preferred by most experienced facial surgeons. It uses the patient's own bone, is very predictable and gives a natural result. Potential complications include nerve injury causing loss of sensation in the lip, which may be permanent. Fortunately, this is extremely rare.

# The operation

Genioplasty is performed under a general anaesthetic. The breathing tube used to ventilate the lungs is normally placed in the nose, allowing the surgeon to work in the mouth unencumbered.

An incision is made in the inside of the mouth, a few millimetres from the lower teeth. The bone of the chin is exposed and care is taken to identify and protect the nerves, which provide sensation to the lip. The lower section of the bone of the chin is separated from the jaw using a drill or saw. This is then advanced and refixed on to the jaw bone using screws or small screws and plates. The wound is then closed, carefully reattaching the muscles of the chin in their original position.

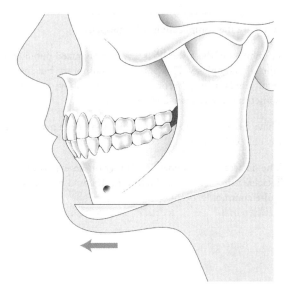

**Figure 11.3** Corrected profile in genioplasty.

Antibiotics are given and the patient is instructed to use an antiseptic mouth-wash for several days. Some swelling is normal but usually settles after about 7–10 days. Any numbness of the lower lip is usually temporary and disappears after a few weeks. The bone heals like any break and takes about 6 weeks. After this, there are no restrictions on physical activity, including contact sports.

## ❓ FAQ

Q 1  What is a chin augmentation?

A  Chin augmentation or augmentation genioplasty describes any procedure that increases the prominence of the chin. This can be achieved in several ways, including the use of fillers, fat or chin implants, or by moving a piece of your own chin bone forwards.

Q 2  When will I see the result?

A  The results of chin augmentation are usually evident immediately after surgery. Swelling in the first week may make the chin look larger than it should be, but this resolves quite quickly.

Q3  What are the complications of genioplasty?

A  Numbness of the lower lip is a well-recognized potential complication of genioplasty. This is usually temporary but may be permanent. Implants may become infected, can move or even be rejected, sometimes many years after surgery.

Q4  I have a large nose and a small chin. Do I need my nose reducing or my chin enlarging?

A  The answer to this depends entirely on an expert analysis of your facial features and skeletal harmony. It could be one or the other or, quite commonly, both!

## *i* Patient's perspective

Alan is a 32-year-old engineer. For several years he has experienced an awareness that he has a 'weak' chin. Although he is not unduly disturbed by this (it is common in most of the men in his family), he thought that a stronger jaw would balance his face and look more masculine.

During a routine annual medical check-up arranged by his employers, he took the opportunity to ask the company doctor about the pros and cons of surgery to improve his chin. The doctor did not feel he could answer all of Alan's questions but offered to refer him to a specialist in cosmetic maxillofacial surgery. Alan took up the referral and attended a consultation with the specialist.

After a general enquiry into his health and previous history, the specialist examined his teeth, jaws, bite, and throat. He took an X-ray of his facial bones and a special X-ray of the lower jaw or mandible called an oral pantomogram. They discussed what Alan was looking for and how it might change his life. The specialist told Alan that there was no underlying problem with his jaws and that his bite or 'occlusion' was normal. He felt that Alan would benefit from a chin augmentation and that his preference was to achieve this by moving the bone of the chin forward, rather than by using an artificial chin implant.

They discussed the possible complications and the surgeon very clearly warned Alan that some alteration of sensation or feeling in the lower lip was a possibility. It was agreed that Alan consider the information he had received and that he would return in a few weeks for a second consultation.

At the second consultation, the specialist showed Alan his X-rays and explained in detail where the bone would be cut. There would be no scars as the incision was to be placed inside the mouth. Alan elected to go ahead and arranged 2 weeks off work to allow for recovery.

The surgery only took an hour and Alan was able to get out of bed and examine his chin in the mirror a few hours after coming round from the anaesthetic. The effect was subtle but at the same time, his whole face seemed to have changed for the better. The following morning, some swelling had increased and the chin looked and felt rather large. This settled down after 4 or 5 days. During this time, Alan had a liquid or soft diet (lots of mashed potato and yoghurt) and carefully rinsed his mouth with an antibacterial mouthwash after every meal. He was instructed to use a very soft toothbrush for at least 2 weeks. For a few days, he noticed a tingling in his lip but no numbness. The cut inside the mouth healed very quickly.

Alan was delighted with the result. Somehow, he felt the surgery had made his face stronger. His family noticed the difference and a few friends thought he was 'better looking'. His brother who had a similar problem went to the same surgeon and had the same operation 6 months later.

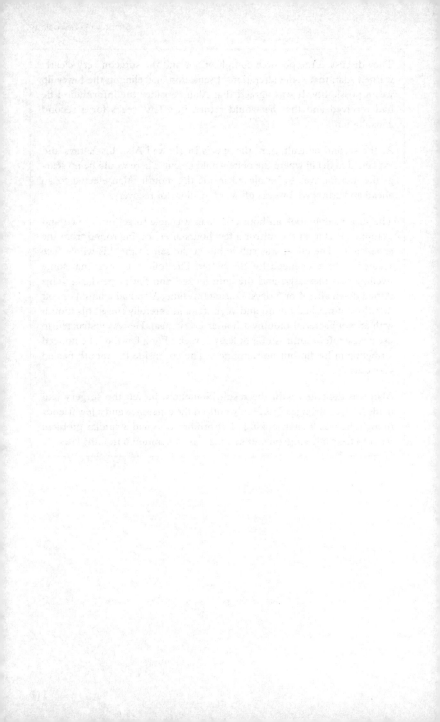

# 12

# Lip surgery

**→ Key points**

- Full plump lips are a desirable feature of a youthful, attractive face.
- Temporary fillers offer a safe, reliable and effective means of enhancing the lip volume.
- Permanent fillers may produce significant complications, even after many years.

Full or plump lips are universally regarded as desirable, attractive, and youthful. They are perceived as sensual and feminine. They have erotic and sexual potential. Lips are enhanced with lipstick and adorned in many cultures, including piercing or stretching with weights.

Ageing can reduce the attractiveness of the lips in many ways. With time, the lips lose volume from a reduction in the glandular tissue and with thinning of the skin. The ridge of tissue at the junction of the mucosa (red lip) and the upper lip skin is called the vermillion border. As this ridge flattens, lipstick may be more difficult to apply and may 'bleed' into any wrinkles formed in the upper lip. With loss of teeth, the bone of the upper jaw also reduces, giving a flatter or even recessed look in the area around the mouth and upper lip. Sun exposure and smoking may also cause deep wrinkles in and around the lip area.

Cosmetic treatment to restore the appearance of a youthful lip is popular and frequently requested. There are many and varied techniques available and while many of them are successful, many women are also anxious that the treatment does not leave them with obvious, artificial, and overinflated lips. Well documented celebrity disasters have heightened this anxiety!

As a general rule, sensible advice for anyone considering lip augmentation is to proceed cautiously and choose injectable fillers that are temporary! In this way, even if the effect is overdone or obvious, there is the comfort of knowing that it will return to normal after a few months.

Hyaluronic acid-based fillers (like Restylane) have many advantages. They are natural products that do not produce allergic responses, are effective in enhancing the lip line and increasing lip volume. Equally, they are gradually resorbed by the body. Although some may see this as a disadvantage, it is comforting to know that any unwanted effect will be temporary. Many patients who have had lip augmentation with permanent fillers are faced with long-term problems if they dislike the result or suffer from any complications, including lumpiness, tissue reaction, allergies, firmness, or pain.

Injection treatments to enhance the lip are usually performed as an outpatient procedure using local anaesthetic. This may be in the form of an anaesthetic cream or injections of local anaesthetic similar to those given at the dentist.

Permanent augmentation can be achieved using the patient's own tissues. These tissues include fat, fascia, or a strip of skin tissue. The advantage is that such tissue will be accepted without rejection, although it may melt away over time. Of the permanent materials available for lip augmentation, a strip of soft silicone can give excellent results, much more natural than some of the other implants that can form tight bands of scar in the lip.

Formal surgical procedures to enhance the lips are less common. However, techniques learned from the treatment of cleft lip and palate can be applied to aesthetic surgery with good results. A thin lip can be improved by advancing tissue from the inside of the lip to increase the volume and fullness. The scars are all hidden inside the mouth. Also, a long lip can be shortened and everted (pouted outwards) using carefully placed scars around the base of the nose.

# 13

# Botox and fillers

## ⮕ Key points

◆ Treatment should only be given by properly trained medical staff.

◆ Understand the difference between permanent and temporary fillers.

◆ Be aware of the potential complications or problems that may occur.

## Botox

The use of Botox to improve appearance has become the most popular 'non-surgical' cosmetic procedure, with about two million patients treated each year in the USA. The word 'Botox' is actually a company trade name for a product containing botulinum toxin. There are currently three other such products with market authorization called Vistabel, Neurobloc, and Dysport.

Botox is derived from a bacteria called *Clostridium botulinum*. This bacterium exists in several forms or types. Type A and B are used in the therapeutic preparations manufactured for human use. Although these bacteria can be responsible for illness in humans, Botox is produced in controlled laboratory conditions and only used in extremely small doses. The amounts of toxin used are much too small to cause any clinical disease.

Botox works by preventing muscles from contracting. It prevents the release of a chemical, acetylcholine, which is necessary to allow nerve impulses to send messages to muscles. Excessive muscle contraction can be responsible for a variety of disorders. These include 'blepharopasm' a condition affecting the eyes, and the flexion contractures that occur in the limbs of children with cerebral palsy. Both these conditions are greatly improved by Botox treatment.

Botox is also used to reduce excessive underarm sweating, for abolishing facial 'tics', and treating anal fissures.

The use of Botox to improve appearance was stimulated by the observations of an ophthalmic surgeon with great experience of treating patients with blepharospasm. It is the contraction of facial muscles that produces lines, wrinkles, and furrows in the skin. These are sometimes referred to as 'dynamic' wrinkles. By preventing muscle contraction, wrinkles and lines can be reduced or abolished.

Botox is used in the face to achieve a smoother, unlined, and fresher appearance. The most popular areas for treatment are the frown lines between the eyebrows and the 'crows feet' at the outer edge of the eyes. In the USA, Botox is now formally approved for cosmetic treatment in this area by the Food and Drug Administration (FDA). It is, however, also used for treating other areas of the face, including the lines around the upper lip and muscle bands in the neck (Figure 13.1).

There are few restrictions on patient's suitability but you should not have Botox if you are:

- pregnant

- breastfeeding

- taking certain antibiotics

- prone to allergies, or

- have a neurological disorder.

The treatment involves administering the Botox by injections with micro-needles. It takes only a few minutes and causes little discomfort. Some redness and swelling may appear at the injection sites but this normally disappears after a few hours.

After treatment, most doctors will advice that you refrain from exercise and alcohol for 24 hours. It may be suggested that you frown or squint as often as possible for several hours after the injections as it is thought to encourage the Botox to fix in the treated area. If the injections damage small veins under the skin, some bruising may result.

The treatment may start to work after a day or two. Often, the area feels 'stiff' for a while. The full effect may take up to 10–12 days to achieve. In the area between the eyebrows, frown lines will disappear. Also, as these muscles lower or depress the brow, weakening them may result in a lifting effect on the whole brow area. Occasionally, this may result in a sharp, excessive arch to the

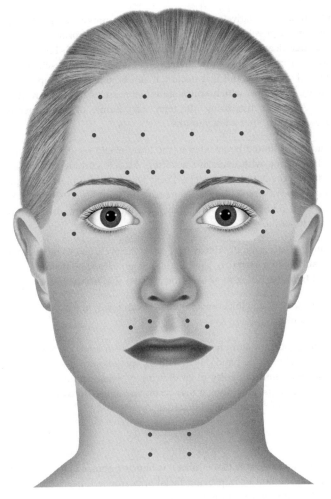

**Figure 13.1** Areas on the face treatable with Botox.

eyebrow or 'mephisto' effect. This can be rectified with further injection of Botox into the brow elevator muscles.

For most people, the effect of Botox is to abolish a tired or angry look and to produce a softer, rested, more youthful appearance.

The effect of the treatment will last for about 4–6 months.

## Complications

Complications are relatively rare and usually of a minor nature. Allergies to the injection are possible but extremely rare. When the eyebrow area is treated, the most significant problem is the 'drooping' of an eyelid. This may occur if the Botox spreads into the eyelid area and paralyses the muscle that opens the eyelid. This is rare and if it occurs, it can be treated with apraclonidine (Iopidone) eye drops, which stimulate other muscles to perform the same function. Although distressing, the temporary nature of Botox means that recovery will occur after a few months.

Botox injection should be avoided in the lower eyelid region as it may cause the eyelid to drop with excessive watering. Muscle contraction can help to pump fluid in the lymphatic system. These lymphatic channels are important in draining extra tissue fluids. By paralysing muscles in the eyelid area, an occasional side-effect of Botox may be a puffy swelling, due to impaired lymphatic function.

As mentioned, occasionally Botox may cause the eyebrows to be raised excessively, resulting in a 'surprised' and unnatural appearance. This can usually be corrected by using Botox to weaken the muscles that lift the brow.

Excessive use of Botox injections in the face can result in a lack of expression or 'frozen' look.

A rare but important complication may result from injecting Botox into the neck to abolish muscle bands. If the Botox spreads into the muscles of the throat, it may cause difficulty in swallowing or even aspiration of food and saliva into the lungs. Therefore, it may be unwise to use Botox for anyone with a neuromuscular or neurological disorder.

# Fillers

The use of injectable soft tissue 'fillers' is hugely popular as it offers a simple non-surgical method of improving facial appearance. They work in a completely different way from Botox.

The basic principle is that plumping, filling, or augmenting tissue can reverse some features of facial ageing, including:

- loss of fullness in the lips

- deepening of the lines that run from the nose to the side of the mouth (the 'nasolabial folds')

♦ lines or wrinkles in the upper lip and other areas of the face

♦ depressions in the skin caused by acne and other scars

♦ a hollow gaunt appearance due to loss of facial fat—this is often seen quite severely in patients treated for HIV infection.

There are a plethora of different types of filler materials. New products are constantly being developed and aggressively marketed to doctors and the public.

## Categories of fillers

### Temporary or resorbable fillers

♦ *Collagen and hyaluronic acid.* These products are popular as they are safe and predictable. Hyaluronic acid fillers in particular, are well tolerated and rarely cause any allergic reaction from the tissues. They are gradually removed or resorbed by the body and last for 2–6 months. The need for repeated injections may be seen as a disadvantage. However, it is also comforting to know that the effects are temporary if the injections are poorly placed or overdone!

♦ *Poly-L-lactic acid.* This is also used as a filler and claims are made that it stimulates the body to produce more of its own collagen. These remain to be substantiated. It is useful when larger volumes are required to replace tissue defects and atrophy, and can last for up to 2 years. It is less useful for very fine lines around the lip and mouth area and may cause some permanent lumpiness due to aggregation of calcium particles.

### Permanent fillers

These products include liquid silicone and a variety of 'micro-implant' materials. These may consist of tiny plastic beads or water-based gels. Although the option of a 'once-only' treatment is enticing, there are well-documented 'downsides' with a range of potential complications. These include:

♦ *Allergic and inflammatory reactions.* These may cause redness, swelling, pain, and lumpiness. An adverse response of this type can be very distressing and difficult to treat. Before treatment with a permanent filler, a skin allergy test is a sensible and often essential requirement.

♦ *Migration.* Over time, the injected material may shift or move from the injection site. Liquid silicone injections are well known for their tendency to move, even after many years.

♦   *Infection and extrusion*. Any foreign material may be prone to infection, which may produce inflamed lumps and abscesses.

In general, the potential for long-term problems should be carefully considered before using these materials.

### Autologous or 'natural' fillers

This category refers to tissues derived from your own body. They include fat, fascia, skin, and even scar tissue. The obvious advantage of using one's own body tissues is that there is no risk of allergy or rejection. Dermis (the deep layer of the skin) is popular for plumping the lips. Facelift operations involve removal of some excess skin and soft tissue from the face. Instead of throwing this away, it is often used to enhance other areas, such as the lip or even the nose.

The first autologous tissue used in cosmetic surgery was fat. Until recently, the problem with fat was its tendency to be resorbed by the body. However, advances in techniques of harvesting and preparing fat have led to a resurgence in its popularity and fat injections are increasingly used to enhance the cheeks, nasolabial lines, and the chin. Improvements in fat survival have been achieved by techniques developed by an American physician, Sidney Coleman. There is currently a great deal of interest in the use of fat transfer to increase the size of the breasts. The option of breast enlargement without implants is obviously appealing. However, the procedure is still unproven and safety concerns have yet to be addressed. These include potential difficulty of interpreting mammograms and the potential of fat cells to be oestrogen-receptor sensitive.

Unfortunately, all autologous tissues can be absorbed by the body over time, and long-term improvement can be difficult to predict.

Recently, there has been a great interest and enthusiasm for using one's own tissue, cultured or grown in the laboratory, for reinjection. However, this is expensive and long-term results have yet to be evaluated. In the UK and the USA, companies producing these tissue derivatives have recently ceased trading!

## The procedure

Injection of fillers of whatever type are usually performed as a simple outpatient procedure. Injection of fillers around the mouth and lips can be painful and usually require some form of local anaesthetic to numb the area. This may include applying a topical cream containing anaesthetic or injecting local anaesthetic, similar to the procedure used by dentists.

After treatment, some redness and swelling may occur in the treated areas. This usually subsides within a day or two.

## Conclusions

Fillers are popular and can be very effective in masking the early signs of ageing in the face. Before treatment, it is essential that the properties and long-term effects of any material are thoroughly explored and any risks are fully explained. It is also important to understand the aims of treatment and the limitations. Although a range of paramedical practitioners act as providers of Botox and fillers, it is worth considering the recommendations of the manufacturers.

> Botox should only be administered by an appropriately qualified physician with experience of facial anatomy and physiology, familiar with the product and the associated equipment.

# appendix

# Useful website resources

**The British Association of Aesthetic Plastic Surgeons (BAAPS)**

http://www.baaps.org

**The British Association of Plastic, Reconstructive and Aesthetic Surgeons**

http://www.bapras.org.uk

**The International Association of Aesthetic Plastic Surgeons**

http://www.isaps.org

**The European Association of Plastic Surgeons**

http://www.euraps.org

**The Royal College of Surgeons of England** has information for patients at

http://www.rcseng.ac.uk

**Medicines and Healthcare Products Regulatory Agency**

www.silicone-review.gov.uk

Further information about breast implants is available from the **Department of Health** website http://www.dh.gov.uk

Independent healthcare providers need to be registered with the **Healthcare Commission.** Registered providers must demonstrate that they meet standards for safety and quality of care, and are assessed regularly. Members of the public can check the Healthcare Commision website to see whether a provider is on the registered list at http://www.healthcarecommission.org.uk

All BAAPS members are on the **Specialist Register of Plastic Surgery.** The General Medical Council holds details of a surgeon's qualifications at http://www.gmc-uk.org

# Glossary

**Abdominal hernia**  A hernia protruding through a defective or weakened portion of the abdominal wall. An umbilical hernia is a type of abdominal hernia.

**Areola**  The brown or pink ring of tissue surrounding the nipple of the breast.

**Autoimmune disease**  One of a group of otherwise unrelated disorders caused by inflammation and destruction of tissues by the body's own immune response. These disorders include rheumatoid arthritis and thyroiditis.

**Blepharitis**  Inflammation of the eyelids.

**Blepharospasm**  Involuntary tight contraction of the eyelids, either in response to painful conditions of the eye or as a form of muscle dysfunction.

**Body mass index**  The weight of a person (in kilograms) divided by the square of the height of that person (in metres); used as an indicator of whether or not a person is over- or underweight.

**Breast asymmetry**  A difference in the size of the breasts.

**Breast implant**  A sac inserted under the skin of the chest wall to restore or improve the shape of the breast.

**Canthopexy**  A condition in which there is a redundancy of the skin of the upper eyelids so that a fold of skin hangs down, often concealing the tarsal margin when the eye is open.
1. An operation for lengthening the palpebral fissure by incision through the lateral canthus. Synonym: cantholysis.
2. An operation for restoration of the canthus.

**Canthus**  The corner of the eye, the angle at which the upper and lower eyelids meet.

**Capsular contracture**  A condition where the implant is invested by tightly woven collagen fibres to form a 'capsule'. Capsules are normal but occasionally the capsule tightens and contracts to produce distortion and shape changes in the breast. This can be painful.

**Columella** The fleshy lower margin (termination) of the nasal septum.

**Cornea** The transparent structure forming the anterior part of the fibrous tunic of the eye.

**Cosmetic surgery** Surgery in which the principal purpose is to improve the appearance, usually with the connotation that the improvement sought is beyond the normal appearance, and its acceptable variations, for the age and the ethnic origin of the patient. Synonym: aesthetic surgery.

**Dermatochalasis** Redundant eyelid skin, usually occurring as a result of ageing.

**Embolism** The sudden blocking of an artery by a clot or foreign material, which has been brought to its site of lodgement by the blood current.

**Haematoma** A localized collection of blood, usually clotted, in an organ, space, or tissue, due to a break in the wall of a blood vessel.

**Liposuction** Removal of body fat from the contours of the body via a suction device.

**Mammogram** A medical investigation to X-ray the breast.

**Mastalgia** Breast pain.

**Mastitis** An infection of the breast, common during breastfeeding.

**Mastopexy** A surgical technique to lift a droopy breast into a more elevated and normal position, often with some improvement in shape.

**Mastopexy/augmentation** A surgical technique where the breast is lifted and an implant placed at the same time.

**Mucosa mucous membrane** The lubricated inner lining of the mouth, nasal passages, vagina, and urethra, or any membrane or lining which contains mucous secreting glands.

**Prostheses and implants** Artificial substitutes for body parts, and materials inserted into tissues for functional, cosmetic, or therapeutic purposes.

**Rectus abdominis** Paired muscles in the abdomen.

**Sclera** The tough white outer coat of the eyeball, covering approximately the posterior five-sixths of its surface and continuous anteriorly with the cornea and posteriorly with the external sheath of the optic nerve.

**Septoplasty** Operation to correct defects or deformities of the nasal septum, often by alteration or partial removal of supporting structures.

**Septorhinoplasty** Combined operation to repair defects or deformities of the nasal septum and of the external nasal pyramid.

**Seroma** A mass or tumefaction caused by the localized accumulation of serum within a tissue or organ.

**Thromboembolism**  Obstruction of a blood vessel with thrombotic material carried by the blood stream from the site of origin to plug another vessel.

**Thrombosis/thrombus**  An aggregation of blood factors, primarily platelets, and fibrin with entrapment of cellular elements, frequently causing vascular obstruction at the point of its formation. Some authorities thus differentiate thrombus formation from simple coagulation or clot formation. Compare with 'embolism'.

# Index